*For Joanna Seymour 1966–2007 and
John Yeatman 1914–2006*

Individualization and the Delivery of Welfare Services

Contents

List of Tables

Preface and Acknowledgements

This book came about as a result of a project on individualized service delivery that was funded by the Australian Research Council 2001–03 to which I offer thanks. I conceived the project and led the project team who included Gary Dowsett, Michael Fine, Diane Gursansky with Joanna Penglase serving as our research officer. Each of these four individuals contributed invaluable and distinctive insights to the project as it unfolded through time even while the normative theoretical vision for the project remained my own.

I have placed a case study from an earlier project I led and conceived (also funded by the Australian Research Council on 'the new contractualism' 1998–2000) in this book because it belongs here: this is Chapter 12 ('Facilitating independence and self-determination: the case of a disability employment service'). This case study originally appeared in 'The Role of Contract in the Democratization of Service Delivery', Anna Yeatman and Kathryn Owler in *Law in Context* 18 (2) 2001, published by Federation Press: www.federationpress.com.au. Thanks are due to Kathryn Owler for sharing the fieldwork for this case study with me.

The conduct of the individualized service delivery project involved a project reference group that met thrice. The group combined policy, practitioner and consumer advocacy expertise as well as commitment to a normative vision for individualized service delivery. The individuals who served on this group gave of themselves generously and creatively. They provided some reality testing for the project; and in the last meeting of the reference group in May 2003, they also indicated that the policy context that had seemed relatively stable at the beginning of the project was changing in such a way as to make the normative orientation of the project seem even more 'heroic' than it had been. I acknowledge the assistance in this project of the following members of the project reference group: Luke Grant, Sheila Ross, Mike Rungie, Sheila Shaver, Phil Tuckerman and Sandy Watson. I acknowledge also the contribution to both team meeting and reference group discussions of Cosmo Howard who at the time of the project's empirical research was undertaking his doctoral dissertation research on Centrelink. In addition, I acknowledge the contributions to team meeting conversation and/or reference group conversations of Carol Austin, Bob McLelland, Bleddyn Davies, Kirsty Machon, John Rule, Rose Melville and Catherine McDonald.

While the project was conceived in Australia and we finished the empirical work we did for the project by the end of 2003, I took much longer figuring out how to theoretically frame the normative vision I had for this project. This was for a number of reasons, not least being how to find my voice as a political theorist in writing about individualization and the welfare state. I undertook this work when I left my position as professor of Sociology at Macquarie University and took up the position as a senior Canada Research Chair in the Department of Political Science, University of Alberta in July 2003. I am grateful for the freedom to engage primarily in research that my holding a Canada Research Chair permitted me. I am grateful also for the Department of Political Science's accession to my wish to focus on advanced graduate seminar teaching for this has grown both me and my ideas. I also benefited from extended theoretical conversations with two young political theorists, Kamila Stullerova and Magdalena Zolkos.

Thanks are due to a number of other individuals who have contributed their insight, vision and experience to this project. These are: Sue Vardon, John Halligan, Levinia Crooks, Michael Hurley, Kane Race, Helen Disney, Elizabeth Morgan, Deidre Cheers, Jude Morwitzer, Craig Unterheiner, Scott Holz, Peta Fitzgibbon, Diana Rose and Gael Fraser.

During the time that this project was theoretically incubating after I had gone to Canada, and between the end of 2003 and the end of 2007, I did the four-year Victoria training in the Feldenkrais Method of somatic education. This training added a practitioner sensibility and awareness to the policy and academic roles I had already acquired. I learnt more than I am able to express from the ethos and ethic of the Feldenkrais Method as it was offered to me by Jeff Haller and Alice Friedman as well as other teachers and my fellow students in the training. This learning overlapped my engagement with post-Kleinian psychoanalytic thinking of the kind associated with the 'Object Relations' tradition, an engagement that has been embedded in my own psychic growth and awareness as facilitated by a generative psycho-therapeutic relationship as a client. There are a number of other people who have contributed to my self-awareness as informally facilitated through the sharing of practices of self awareness: Catherine Kellogg, David Kahane, Cressida Heyes, Mridula Nath Chakraborty, David Levine, Sasha Roseneil and Paul Hoggett.

During the time that I was theoretically digesting the project in Canada my father and my oldest niece died. Both of these losses have been hard for me. I especially grieve my niece's death given that she was only 40 when she died, and I had only just got to know her in an adult way. Each of these two individuals was a professional deeply and intelligently committed to individualized service delivery: my father as a general practitioner, my niece as principal of a primary school in a working class area of Adelaide. The dedication of the book to them is to honor the prideful tradition of a passionate civic professionalism oriented to the public good that these two individuals represent. This is a tradition I associate with many people I have had the pleasure and good fortune to know especially if not only in Adelaide, South Australia where my own subjective formation occurred.

I wish my niece could have read this book; with her incisive, no-holds-barred and passionate intelligence, she would certainly have improved it. I was lucky to have two discerning readers for the theoretical part of the book: Deirdre Croft, an Australian mother of a severely intellectually handicapped adult son, a trained journalist, a disability advocate, and someone who is completing a PhD on Accommodation Support for Western Australians with Intellectual Disability; and Magdalena Zolkos, a political theorist, Polish by origin, who works in the field of transitional justice and reconciliation.

As I send this book to press, I am aware of another set of changes in my life. In July 2008 I move from Edmonton, Canada to take up the new position of foundation director and professor of a new research centre at the University of Western Sydney: the Centre for Citizenship and Public Policy.

Anna Yeatman

Notes on Contributors

Gary W. Dowsett
Gary Dowsett, PhD, is Professor and Deputy Director at the Australian Research Centre in Sex, Health and Society at La Trobe University in Melbourne. He is also an Associate Professor of Clinical Sociomedical Sciences at Columbia University in New York. A sociologist, he has worked on sexuality research, particularly in relation to the rise of modern gay communities. Since 1986, he has been researching the HIV epidemic, particularly in Australia's gay communities, and has worked on many international HIV/AIDS and sexual health projects since the late 1980s. He has recently been developing training programs in community-based research and qualitative research design. His book *Practicing Desire: Homosexual Sex in the Era of AIDS* was published by Stanford University Press in 1997.

Michael D. Fine
Michael D. Fine is Associate Professor in Sociology and Deputy-Director, Centre for Research on Social Inclusion, at Macquarie University, Sydney. His current and recent research concerns the sociology of care and human services, addressing theories of and international developments in care, globalization, demography and carework, links between formal and informal support, individualization and social isolation, and innovative patterns of service delivery. His book *A Caring Society? Care and the Dilemmas of Human Service in the Twenty-First Century* was published by Palgrave Macmillan in 2007.

Diane Gursansky
Diane Gursansky is a Senior Lecturer in the School of Social Work and Social Policy at the University of South Australia. She maintains a strong practice base in her profession of social work. She is the co-author with Judy Harvey and Rosemary Kennedy of *Case Management: Policy, Practice and Professional Business* (Allen & Unwin, Crows Nest, Australia, 2003). Her research interests include: service delivery, particularly case management and design of service delivery systems; social work practice; aged care; field education; and evaluation research. She has held Ministerial appointments on the Social Security Appeals Tribunal and currently sits on the Child Death and Serious Injury Committee in South Australia.

Joanna Penglase

Joanna Penglase is the co-founder of Care Leavers Australia Network (CLAN) the Sydney-based national support and advocacy body for care survivors. CLAN was instrumental in establishing the Senate Inquiry into Children in Institutional Care. Dr Penglase has had a long career in research: firstly in documentary film production and then in academic research, particularly in the area of child protection and out of home care. In 2005 she published *Orphans of the Living Growing Up in 'Care' in Twentieth-Century Australia* (Curtin University Books/Fremantle Press, republished 2007), the only published work on this history in Australia, and in 2007 she was awarded the Order of Australia Medal for her work as an advocate for care survivors. She continues to work with CLAN in an administrative, advocacy and research capacity.

Anna Yeatman

Anna Yeatman was a senior Canada Research Chair (Social Theory and Policy) in the Department of Political Science, University of Alberta until mid-2008 when she took up the position as Director of the Centre for Citizenship and Public Policy, University of Western Sydney. She regards herself as an interdisciplinary political theorist interested in contemporary liberal-republican conceptions of the state, personhood, citizenship, and subjective life. She has done a number of Australian-based consultancies in public policy, the last of which was the review of the First Commonwealth-State Disability Agreement (1995–6) that issued in two reports. She completed a training in the Feldenkrais Method in 2007.

Part I

Theoretical Perspectives on Individualization and the Delivery of Welfare Services

Anna Yeatman

1
Introduction

The status aspect of individualization

In any social organization people are situated in relation to each other in terms of their respective status. Status concerns how someone is ethically valued by others—whether they are considered equal, superior, inferior; whether they are considered worth listening to or not; whether they are regarded as exemplifying the best or the worst, the sacred or the profane, in a particular type of society. Individualization is a term that can mean different things. Here it is used with reference to the status of people, that is, people considered in the ethical aspect of their relationship to other people. Individualization considered in its status aspect refers to the equal entitlement of each human being to be considered a subject of right or, as Hegel (1991) put it, a person.

Individualization denotes an ethical ordering of human relationships that is associated with a modern type of society, where the individual rather than the group (the domestic group or some other kind of group modelled after kinship bonds) is constituted and valued as the unit of social action. In an individualized type of society, relationships between people are structured and thought about so that they become open and responsive to the individuals who participate in them.[1] For this to occur, people have to understand what it is to be considered an individual, to develop the capabilities that permit them to act as individuals, and to recognize their fellow participants in social life as individuals. When it is the individual who acquires this ethical status in the organization of social life, groups have to structure their existence so that they honour the status of those who are considered individuals.

The idea of the individual as the subject of right

The idea of the individual as the subject of right is an ethical artefact. That is, according to each human being the status of a person depends on a societal valuing of individuality or of an individual's freedom to live life in his or her own way. It is as an individual that a human being is invited to engage in the challenge of living his or her life as someone who is free to consider how s/he wishes to do this.

Subjective right is the term I will use for the ethical conception of each human being as one who ought to enjoy the status of an individual or person. As I explain in this book the only conception of individual freedom that fits an inclusive and universal idea of subjective right is that which belongs to the individual considered as a self. Freedom in this frame of reference refers to the freedom of the self to assume life in such a way that it is expressive of his or her integrity as a self. As I show, freedom so understood can be enjoyed by babies and children and by people with relatively severe levels of cognitive impairment; it does not have to be reserved for cognitively competent adult subjects.

Two competing conceptions of the individual as the subject of right

There is an alternative conception of individual freedom, one that is associated with the idea of the will. In this frame of reference, an individual is free if s/he is able to will for him or herself, that is, to make decisions for him or herself under conditions where it can be assumed that this individual has sufficient cognitive competence and information to make self-responsible and rationally sensible decisions. I do not discount the importance of such competence for autonomous decision making, but I argue two things. First, the freedom to make choices and decisions for oneself is genuine freedom only if the subject concerned has an autonomous sense of self that finds expression in these choices and decisions. This consideration is usually ignored by those who champion the idea of freedom as a freedom of choice. The telling question is the one that David Levine (see Levine 1995, 24–29) asks, how does an individual know that his or her choices/preferences are his or her own as distinct from what it is that others want him or her to choose or want? Thus, on the principle that the more inclusive conception is better than the less inclusive one, the idea of the self as the subject of freedom is more adequate than the idea of the will as the subject of freedom. Secondly, as already suggested, freedom expressed as the capacity to will for oneself is the old idea of freedom understood in terms of the capacity for self-government. As Aristotle put it, someone who can govern himself can govern others. This is clearly a discriminatory idea of freedom for it excludes all human beings who, for whatever reason, cannot govern themselves from the status entitlement to conduct their life as a free person. This is an obvious issue in the domain of welfare services for, as we shall see, welfare services concern the fate of people whose capacity for self-government is either non-existent, impaired, or currently compromised by abjection of one kind or another. To put it slightly differently, the idea of the will cannot be reconciled with the idea of the individual in an inclusive and non-discriminatory conception of human rights (see Yeatman 2001).

Contemporary welfare debate as conflict between the idea of the subject of right as a self or as a will

These, then, are two different and conflicting frameworks for thinking about the status of the individual as the subject of right, as a person. This is not an academic observation of the kind that has no practical implication. I argue in this book that our contemporary welfare debate is structured as a conflict between these two frameworks for thinking about individualization in its ethical import. As we shall see, while one framework (that of the self as the subject of right) indicates an expansive public welfare state where attention must be given to the question of service delivery, the other framework (that of the will as the subject of right) indicates a minimalist public welfare state where the question of service delivery does not assume any particular salience.

Welfare is a term that means the same thing as well-being. Well-being refers to anything that conduces to the life and integrity of the subject whose well-being is at issue. The integrity of the will is not the same thing as the integrity of the self. The idea of welfare is quite different depending on which of these ideas of the individual as the subject of right is in play. It is important to understand what is at stake here for, without such understanding, it is impossible to intelligently engage with the current terms of the debate about public responsibility for welfare services.

If it can be argued that welfare services are a fundamental condition of the possibility of human subjects getting to be effective or actual selves in their life worlds, then the argument is one of proposing that the right to personhood demands of the state that it provide welfare services that, among other things, make this right possible. The conception of the subjective right of the individual considered as a self as the basis of social policy is an argument that has not been elaborated in theoretical conceptions of the welfare state. If such argument has been neglected theoretically, it has not been neglected within the practical world of welfare services. There we find many practitioners and the professional educators of practitioners eloquently voicing a conception of welfare services that respond to the needs of the human subject considered as a self. Some of the more considered of those who write about this conception rightly emphasize its complexity (e.g. Davis 2001; McCormack 2002; Sinason 1992). Also in these practical worlds we find self-advocates, people who communicate how they need welfare services if they are to enjoy freedom to live their lives in such a way that it articulates their self experience (I owe this term to Bollas 1993).

The right to self-preservation as the basis of a conception of welfare

In work I have done as an evaluator of two major collaborative program initiatives shared across the Australian federal and state/territory governments, I have heard self-advocates put their case with a crystal clear understanding of how welfare services designed in such a way as to respond to their sense of self makes it possible for them to be a person. The more I thought about it, I could find no ready-to-hand theoretical conception that could philosophically account for these practical conceptions. At some point in this enquiry, I realized that I could open up the seventeenth century conception of a right to self-preservation if I asked one simple question: what is this idea of the self that deserves to be preserved (see Yeatman 2007b)? From this point on, I could integrate my experience of welfare services both as they have been written about by practitioners and by self-advocates with a theoretical explication of the individual subject of right as a self.

The seventeenth century conception is one of a *right* to self-preservation. It is, thus, a specification of the ethical standing of the individual considered as a being with its own integrity and uniqueness. Seventeenth century civil philosophy of the kind we associate with John Locke and other thinkers is oriented to enquiry into how social relationships need to be ordered as civil relationships that make it possible for each human being to enjoy the standing of someone who has a right to self-preservation (see

Yeatman 2009). In seventeenth century civil philosophy, the unit of social organization that attends to the welfare of most individuals is the patriarchal household, but the civil standing of the heads of such households as individual subjects of right, as persons, is secured by the sovereign authority of the state under law. Accordingly, in this framework welfare did not assume the aspect of a civil project. This could occur only once the authority of the patriarchal household had lost legitimacy, and the question of how all the status of all human beings considered as each a subject of right entered into the political question of security for each person's welfare. It is in this context that I argue we can revisit the idea of a right to self-preservation and turn it into the basis of a civil project of welfare.

The right of each individual as a self to welfare and its implications for service delivery

In arguing for a conception of welfare services that facilitate, assist with and support an effective sense of self on behalf of those who need them, I show how this conception of welfare services must lead to concern with service delivery: with the relationship of service delivery, with the quality of service delivery, and with how good and effective service delivery needs to be facilitated and supported by the state as the public authority responsible for ensuring that welfare services function on behalf of the right of each human subject to self-preservation. It is only the state as the sovereign authority under law that can articulate and uphold a public set of expectations and norms concerning what it is to share ethical life as a plurality of individuals, each entitled to subjective right.

Without clarifying the terms of their case, it is difficult for proponents of this conception of welfare services to have the influence over the terms of welfare debate that they deserve. All the case studies selected for this book are illuminating and contextually-specific stories of practical experimentation in welfare services that are oriented to the claims of the self. These examples of imaginative and creative institution building on behalf of welfare services are taken from the Australian context from 1996–2003. They were developed within a policy environment that had been remarkably stable from mid-1970s onwards. However at the point at which we constructed these case studies, the policy environment had already begun to shift from one that was oriented to the person considered as a self to one that was oriented to the person considered as a will.

As I have said, the will is an older conception of the individual, one that is not only exclusive of children and of people whose cognitive impairment means that they cannot be regarded as able to govern themselves. It excludes also adults who are cognitively capable but who, for some reason, do not actualize their potential for private property ownership, a potential that resides in their ability to sell their capacity to labour in the modern employment market, and to gain an income in exchange for this sale. Effective exercise of the will, then, demands not just adult mental competence but also the individual's private ownership of property for the individual accesses services, welfare services among these, through trading his or her property for them (s/he purchases them). In this conception of welfare, those who lack either one or both of these two aspects of the effective will—adult mental competence, private wealth—are uneasily positioned in relation to this idea of personhood; they cannot really be regarded as subjects of right, and, accordingly, they have no entitlement to public welfare services. Instead, the rationale for such public welfare services as they may receive involves any one or combination of the following: (a) an argument that these people should be induced or forced into the subjective comportment of the disciplines of the will; (b) they are worthy objects of the charity of the beneficent will; and (c) to the extent they present a public nuisance, they have to be managed, and, if necessary, segregated and/or incarcerated.

This is not a conception of welfare services designed to facilitate the sense of self of the client. Instead, public welfare services are regarded instrumentally, as a means to a societal end that is external to the service transaction in question. The same instrumental logic governs the idea of the private purchase of welfare services. As will, the individual is positioned as a consumer of welfare services; s/he asserts his or her will in relation to the agent from whom s/he is purchasing the service. His or her will not only drives the transaction but exists prior to the service delivery relationship which, accordingly, is placed as a means to the realization of his or her will as its end. The instrumental conception of the delivery of welfare services discounts the significance of the welfare professional's autonomy for the creation of a safe and relatively insulated space within which the welfare service delivery relationship can be built and function.

The intention guiding this book

The primary intention guiding this book is one of clarifying an ethical conception of welfare services as services designed to secure an inclusive and non-discriminatory conception of subjective right at a time when this conception has faltered. It is not just that government has drifted away from this conception with more or less deliberate ideological intent, but those who are passionate proponents of the claims of the self in relation to welfare services have lost a public voice. With the abandonment of a welfare policy that is oriented to subjective right, government has made it seem that the new policy direction is more 'modern' than the old one, and they discredit the proponents of what now seems the 'old' way of doing things as naïve and behind the times. Such rhetoric depends on a technological conception of welfare as a set of causal relationships which can be known, and made subject to knowledge or evidence-based intervention. The essential problem with such thinking is that it positions the subject of welfare as an object of technological mastery, as a thing rather than as a self.

A note on the use of the term 'welfare services'

Unless otherwise indicated, when I use the term 'welfare services' I am referring to all services designed to develop and secure the sense of self of the individual. Such services can include educational and health services. In fact the boundaries between welfare, health and education services can be blurred. On many occasions, a 'welfare' service, for example a service designed to assist someone with a mental illness to develop life management skills is also a teaching-and-learning (thus educational) relationship. So too are health services when they are more than a technical event (diagnostic testing, surgery, pharmacological treatment) and involve a complex dialogue between clinician and client that weighs different kinds of information and value in relation to how best to attend to this client's health needs (for example see Chapter 11).

Welfare services oriented to the needs of the self

Welfare services here are services that make the difference to whether an individual is able to assume life as a self. By assuming life as a self, I mean different things: (a) being accorded dignity and recognition as a unique centre of subjective life whose sense of self must enter into how the service in question is specified and delivered; (b) being facilitated and assisted in an independence or freedom of action that expresses the individual's intentional existence as a self, one whose active mode of being expresses her desires; and (c) being facilitated and assisted in the development of self-awareness, a capacity to reflect on one's subjective experience, on possibilities for self-existence that can be explored, and on what it is one needs to learn in order to assume responsibility for one's own inner life so that one does not project one's own emotional difficulties onto others.

There are many people who are deeply dependent on welfare services, meaning that if they do not get access to welfare services that assist these individuals in assuming life as a self, their self-preservation is at risk. By this we mean not so much that they may risk death through failure to assist them with their needs, although this could and does occur. Rather we mean that without such welfare service assistance and facilitation, these individuals cannot enjoy the freedom of being a self whose life in a significant way is shaped by his or her sense of self.

The people we have in mind here include the following: older people who have become frail and who cannot continue to practice an independence of action that permits them to live intentionally as a self who can satisfy his or her desires, but who can do so with welfare service assistance; people with a cognitive impairment who cannot achieve an effective sense of self without welfare service assistance; young adults whose sense of self is damaged in some way, meaning that they experience difficulty in functioning independently (taking care of themselves, making a living, reflecting on what it is that they want and following lines of action that enable them to fulfil their wants, and engaging in self-nourishing personal relationships), but whose growth as someone who can do these things can be facilitated and assisted by appropriate welfare services; and people suffering a chronic and life-threatening illness that brings about profound feelings of loss, fear, abjection, and vulnerability, but who can engage in a self-determined relationship to how they live with their illness with appropriate assistance and support from welfare services.

If our sight is on welfare services that make the difference to whether people have effective entitlement to self-preservation or not, it is important to extend our conception of the range of such services beyond those that seem obviously urgent such as the provision of home care to a frail, older individual who is at risk of falling and seriously injuring herself without such assistance or the provision of HIV-AIDS drug treatments to someone who is HIV-positive or the provision of out-of-home care to children who have been removed from their parental home. For there are many welfare services that make a difference to whether people get to feel that they are living an existence that is shaped by their needs as a self or not. Consider, for example, women who stay at home to care for a severely disabled child. These mothers can survive without service assistance although their health may suffer, and they may neglect the needs of their other children; but how far can their sense of self be intact, alive, or functional, if these individuals feel that the responsibility of care that they have voluntarily undertaken has turned into an unremitting prison sentence? Consider also young adults who find themselves struggling to learn to manage and live with mental illness. Whether they get to feel they are living an existence that is shaped by their needs as a self depends on whether the psychiatric services they depend on are oriented to and work with their sense of self, whether there are community-based support services that assist them in averting psychotic episodes, and learning to live with their illness, whether there is public income and housing support that ensure they do not have to live in the streets, and so on. Consider also parents who are struggling with how damage to their respective sense of self causes them to fail their children in ways that will damage their children's sense of self but where all of these individuals—the parents as well as the children—could learn to interact in ways that honour and esteem the distinct self that each of them are with appropriate facilitation and assistance from a welfare service. Or domestic partners who find themselves in a vicious cycle of self-abuse and abuse of the other but who can learn to take responsibility for their own conduct, and interact more positively, openly, and reflectively, with appropriate welfare assistance and facilitation.

We could keep on adding examples of services that make a difference to whether people feel they are living an existence that is shaped by their needs as a self or not. Think of settlement services for immigrants that assist them in learning how to adapt to a new social, cultural, and governmental context in ways that do not require them to abandon a sense of self that was formed in a different place, culture, and governmental frame of conduct; or services for refugees; or services designed to assist with the recognition of overseas qualifications for newly arrived immigrants. Or rape counselling services; or services designed to assist young people in making informed and self-regarding decisions regarding their sexual activity. The important thing is to be clear as to the conception of welfare services we have in mind: *these are welfare services that function on behalf of the needs of the individual considered as a self.*

Some of these welfare services are recent developments—rape counselling and drug and alcohol counselling services for example. Others are extensions of older established systems of social security, health and welfare services. This is no accident for the twentieth century elaboration of welfare services can be understood only when viewed in terms of the individual's entitlement to self-preservation. The difficulty, however, with the idea of self-preservation is that it tends to be taken for granted at least in most of the established constitutional democracies such as those associated with Britain, Australia, Scandinavia, the Netherlands, and France. In these contexts it is assumed that of course older people who need help in order to live should get it. It takes a moment to recognize that this is a normative assumption that is not at all obvious. Rather it depends on a societal valuing of the individual who is this older person in need of help that becomes articulated as a public responsibility of the state. If it took until the twentieth century in societies like Britain and Australia for the older person to be seen as a legitimate claimant on welfare services that assisted this individual in continuing to live, then we should ask why, what shifted or became more elaborated in the idea of the welfare subject to make this development seem important or necessary? I discuss this further in Chapter 2.

The subject of welfare as contested terrain

The development of welfare services so conceived under the sponsorship of the state has been uneven, contradictory (advances in their development have been stymied or even simply stopped by changes in government policy), and, as a general rule, under-funded. So if this new conception of welfare services has developed, it does not seem to have met with public consensus. This is a complex topic, but there is one aspect of it I shall discuss here. The normative conception of the human being as an individual entitled to self-preservation is neither well understood nor is it consensual. These two issues—lack of adequate understanding of this ethical value and lack of consensus on it— are surely linked. For if the ethical conception of self-preservation is largely neglected in discussion of the rights of the individual and how they should influence our idea of welfare services, then this may be because a clear idea of self-preservation would expose the lack of consensus concerning the centrality of this idea.

Logically, the right to self-preservation should precede all other rights (I elaborate on this point in Chapter 3). In other words, civil or political rights make sense if they elaborate a pre-existing freedom, the freedom to assume life in society as a self who is entitled to shape her life and relationships so that they express her sense of self. What we find in the history of the modern society is a persistent debate concerning the question of subjective right: is it to be understood in terms of the integrity of the self or as the right to own private property (the freedom of the will)? As Jennifer Nedelsky (1990) has shown for the history of the United States constitutional settlement, property right was permitted a primordial status in relation to all other rights. In seventeenth century civil philosophy of the kind we associate with the thought of John Locke, ownership of property was conceived as expressive of the right to self-preservation; and John Locke drew the logical conclusion that property right could not trump the right to self-preservation.[2] Property right requires that the individual as the subject of right assume existence as a unilateral will free to master and command what it owns. A public ethic of property right requires that individual property owners reciprocally recognize each other's private right to do lawfully what they will with what it is that they own. The problem with property right is that it cannot effectively acknowledge the right to self-preservation of the individuals who come within the private jurisdiction of an individual's property right. They may be his wife, his employees or his children, but on the basis of property right, his respect for their right to self-preservation is contradicted by his right to do as he wills with his own.[3]

Exposure of this difficulty—the failure of property right to secure the right to self-preservation on a non-discriminatory and inclusive basis—is not new (it is one of the central points that Marx and the Labour movement made). It is not remedied by the extension of property right to women so that they are constituted as fully possessive of wills of their own. Yet while this difficulty is at times exposed, most of the time the difficulty in reconciling these two kinds of right is fudged so that it does not have to be faced. While the adoption of human rights discourse in mid-twentieth century international law has influenced the domestic law of the constitutional state societies we have in view—Britain, Australia, Canada, for example—the investment in keeping human rights rhetoric more of a sentimental humanitarian discourse than a closely specified elaboration of an inclusive right to self-preservation is considerable.

To briefly recapitulate this point, property right endows the individual property owner with a will that he is entitled to exercise unilaterally over that which is said lawfully to belong to his private jurisdiction or *dominium*. Over that which he owns, he has the right of mastery: he can do with it what he wills. Even though the older idea of the father owning his children as his property (or chattels as the eighteenth century jurist Blackstone put it) no longer commands legitimacy, when the idea of property right is in play and the individual is accorded standing as a will free to impose itself unilaterally, it is difficult to see how such an individual can be a parent who is able to recognize his child as a separate, distinct, and unique being with needs, desires, and thoughts of her own.

When the subject imagines him or herself as a will that ought to know what s/he wants, that ought to be able to get what s/he wills, and that ought to have enough wealth to buy what s/he wants, these are not the claims of the self but the claims of the will. In this way of thinking about oneself as a subject, relations with equals are conceived as relationships between wills. What cannot be encompassed by way of consciously planned sequences of will-directed action has to fall outside the will's purview. As will, then, the individual cannot know much of the dynamics of his or her inner life for these are generally not within his or her conscious control. Feelings that do not fit his or her image of a self-disciplined individual—an individual who uses the freedom of the will to rule or govern him/herself—have to be disavowed, especially feelings of abjection, vulnerability, and dependency. This is an individual who has difficulty coming to claim and know his or her needs as a self, or as a centre of subjective life. Accordingly, s/he must have difficulty in welcoming, inviting, and recognizing others to be present with him or her as the needy selves that they are. Need, in this framework, is pejoratively reduced to the expression of neediness, understood as compromising rather than as expressive of the freedom to be an individual.

When the idea of the individual that is in play is that of the will, the individual attempts to split off aspects of their being that they cannot reconcile with the ideal of self-government understood as self-mastery. They project these feelings onto other individuals who seem to exemplify the kind of failure of will that is associated with dramatic examples of vulnerability, abjection and dependency: the homeless person who may be also addicted to drugs or alcohol, and who seems to bear on their being the most fearful marks of dereliction. On the other hand, where the idea of the individual that is in play is that of the self, there is nothing incongruent about accepting that this is a self who may have feelings of vulnerability, abjection and dependency, but who can learn to express these feelings in a self-responsible way—one that takes responsibility for expressing, exploring and coming to own these feelings in such a way that is respectful of the existence of others as separate selves.

The debate concerning the idea of welfare services

The idea of welfare services has to be shaped by a normative conception of the individual as the subject of need. I have introduced two distinct and conflicting normative ideas of the individual as the subject of need: the individual as will; the individual as a self. It turns out, then, that we cannot use a single reference to the term 'individualization' in relation to welfare services. We need to be clear about which conception we wish to adopt.

With the idea of the individual as will, there is inherent difficulty in reconciling the notion of success in being this kind of individual with need. Success as this kind of individual is expressed in the achievement of the disciplines of the will as these are manifest in individual ownership of private property. Need is accommodated in this framework, so far as it is accommodated at all, either as the need of the self-reliant individual who has sufficient private property to provide for her own needs by purchasing services in the market economy; or as the need of individuals who, for reasons of developmental immaturity (they are children), cognitive impairment (they have an intellectual disability, a brain injury, or dementia), or of failing powers in old age, cannot achieve the disciplines of the will. In this normative framework, there is little legitimacy for welfare provision to meet the need of adults who are not old and frail, and who do not suffer cognitive impairment, unless it is clear that their inability to self-reliantly provide for their own welfare has come about through no fault of their own. So in this framework, for example, in the Australian context, government provision of drought assistance to offset financial losses to farmers is an acceptable form of income support, as is the provision of an old age pension; but government provision of income support to unemployed people, who it is assumed could work if only they had the will to, is viewed as morally problematic.

When this framework governs 'welfare reform'—as it has in the most recent waves of 'welfare reform' (see Mead and Beam 2005), in the United States, in Britain, and in Australia—it leads to policy intended to achieve two things. Firstly, recreate the logic of the 1834 British Poor Law, by so designing the provision of public income support that there are built-in disincentives for people either coming onto or staying on income support. In reference to US welfare reform of the 1990s, Lawrence Mead calls this 'diversion': '[i]n part, reform demanded work simply by driving off the roles families that could support themselves, or by deterring them from coming on'. He comments further on the same page:

> In this understanding, rights to welfare are balanced by the rights of other people. Through the criminal law, government requires that citizens respect the rights and properties of others. Similarly,

diversion, requires that welfare claimants respect the taxpayers, who fund their aid. At least for claimants with alternatives, the policy aims to restore the situation before the welfare state, where people were forced to labor simply by necessity (Mead 2005, 174).

Secondly, for people 'who have no alternative to going on aid, at least in the short term' (Mead 2005, 175), provide public income support in such a way that it is conditional on their willingness to work, and, to find employment that can provide a more legitimate source of income to support themselves: 'Recipients must enter programs, perhaps prepare for work through training, and then look for work (Mead 2005, 175)'. Here we can see at work the logic of a paternalistic individualization, the idea that people must be forced into the disciplines of the will associated with self-reliant 'adult' action. Thus, the conception of the individual as will licenses, and indeed requires, a distinction between 'the deserving' and 'the undeserving' with reference to the public provision of welfare services to adults.

The idea of forcing people into the disciplines of the will associated with achieving self reliance through employment is not normally associated with an emphasis on service delivery, although there are exceptions. Lawrence Mead (1997) explicitly defends a 'new paternalism' or supervisory approach to the management of the poor. He argues for government intervention in actively reshaping the behaviour of welfare recipients (see for discussion of this Yeatman 2000), and, where necessary, for an intensive type of 'personalized' case management approach to poor adults dependent on income support. However, within an essentially instrumental approach to welfare reform, it is easy for government expenditure on personalized programs of behaviour management to be displaced by one that is allegedly more efficient in managing people's behaviour: show us you are looking for work, or be punished, punishment being either forfeiture of income support for a stipulated period of time, or in the event of sustained non-compliance with the rules, being deemed ineligible for income support.

When it is the individual as a self who is considered the subject of welfare, how service delivery functions becomes a prominent set of issues. Considered as a self, the individual is entitled to have his or her sense of self or subjective experience taken seriously by those with whom s/he interacts. In the world of welfare services, this means that both the 'what' and the 'how' of the service need to be oriented to the individual considered as a unique centre of subjective experience. Specifically, and as needed, welfare service provision for individuals con-

sidered as selves should be designed to do any one or more of the following: (a) facilitate the individual's presence as a self in his or her relationships by listening to his or her way of communicating his or her
sense of self, even if s/he cannot use words, and by including what is of
subjective importance to him or her in the 'what' and 'how' of the
welfare service; (b) facilitate and assist in the individual's acquisition
and maintenance of capacities for independent action, there being no
contradiction here in the provision of assistance on which the individual is dependent in order to be independent (as in for example the
daily provision of assistance with transfer from bed to wheelchair, toi-
leting, washing oneself, and transportation from home to work);
(c) facilitate and assist in the individual's development of a self-aware
relationship to his or her being. This involves growing the individual's
capacity to think about his or her subjective experience so that s/he is
able to: clarify what it is that s/he wants; open up possibilities of new
ways of engaging his or her self that past habitual patterns of adaptation to what others have seemed to want of him or her shut down;
work through past injuries, trauma and damage to the self by being
supported in coming to terms with his or her pain and sense of loss
in relation to them; know, as distinct from seeking not to know, the
'dark' side of inter-subjective relationships and assume responsibility
for his or her own conduct both towards him or her self and other
selves; and achieve an acceptance of him or her self on the basis of
which s/he can continue to learn and grow as someone taking up the
challenge of being alive as the self that s/he is and able to call others
alive as selves (this idea of calling the self into aliveness I take from
Alvarez 2002).

When welfare services are oriented to the self, the relationship
between service deliverer and the individual client assumes an importance that it would not otherwise. The 'what' of service provision is
not unimportant; in fact it is central to whether the individual's needs
are met. Consider again an individual's needs for daily personal care.
Yet if personal care is provided in such a way that it does not respond
to the needs of the individual as a self—how this individual likes to be
touched and spoken with, how his or her already achieved expertise in
collaborating with a past personal carer needs to be drawn upon in
working with a new one, where s/he likes his or her things to be put
and so on—then it dishonours the individual's sense of self. Not only
that, if personal care is provided in an industrial manner, treating the
task at hand as a simple means-end calculus, the client is treated as a
thing—something to be managed. Hegel (1991) offers a provocative

concept of what is a thing as distinct from a subject: a thing is something that is 'external' to the subject, thus something that is not mediated by the principle of subjectivity. Being treated as a thing rather than as a subject is likely to arouse in the individual client alarm concerning her safety and resistance. It is much less secure a way of meeting the individual's needs than one that works with his or her sense of self and draws upon his or her self experience and competences.

If service delivery is not structured as an inter-subjective relationship between selves, a situation is created where it is easy to discount or damage the needs of not just the client but also the service worker. In his defence of a republican conception of the entitlement to the status of individuality—being recognized as an individual whose sense of self is to be honoured in the conduct of relationships—Philip Pettit (2002, 342) proposes that relationships must be conducted so that 'the avowed or readily avowable interests' of the individual can be tracked. If they are not tracked, then, it is all too easy for the individual client to be exploited, dominated, abused, simply neglected or disregarded by the service worker. The only way the interests (needs, wishes, desires) of the individual can be tracked, so that they inform the 'what' and the 'how' of the service, is if the service relationship is so structured that the service worker has time, opportunity, permission and skill to listen to how the individual 'avows' his or her interests. Again, this does not mean the individual in question has to be able to use words. I remember a severely demented woman living with her husband, both Polish immigrants living in Adelaide, South Australia, whom I met in 1989 when I went around with her domiciliary care worker on a day she was seeing her clients.[4] This woman's mind was almost completely gone and it would be all too easy to treat her as though she were no longer a subject; yet as the worker reflected with me, this was someone who still showed animation in relation to her husband's presence. The service conundrum in this case was how to provide her husband with much needed respite care without causing severe alarm to his wife, finding herself in strange surroundings with strange people. I cannot remember the solution or if there was one; but my point is that her avowed or readily avowable interests were tracked in how this service was delivered to her and to her husband.

The question of whether the client's avowed or readily avowed interests are tracked in the design and delivery of a particular service is in principle determinable by a third party, charged with undertaking public responsibility for this kind of oversight of service delivery (e.g. an Ombudsman or Auditor-General or government agency responsible

for implementation of human rights legislation within a particular jurisdiction). This is an important way of making service delivery accountable to a public ethic of subjective right.

If the service worker is to respond to the self of the service client,
then the worker needs to feel valued as a self. If the policy environment of the service delivery relationship bureaucratizes the service
delivery relationship by subjecting it to externally prescribed rules, procedures, and form-filling that deprive the service worker of initiative,
creativity, and, above all, a sense of being trusted to respond professionally and appropriately to the needs of the individual client, then
the service worker's sense of self is discounted. If the service delivery
agency environment is resource-straitened, and stressed, there being
no provision for the training and supervision of workers, and, instead,
individual workers carry the can for policy, program and agency failure, then the service worker risks damage and injury to her sense of
efficacy as a self in this capacity. If the client is positioned in a market
relationship to an individual worker—the client has bought the worker's
service—then, unless there is third party oversight of the relationship
to ensure that both client's and worker's interests inform the framing
and conduct of the relationship, it is all too easy for the client to assume
the prerogative of the propertied will in relation to her employee, and
treat the worker as simply an instrument to fulfil her will. While this
might seem the only way to operate for those who identify with being
an individual *qua* will, there is no provision in this arrangement for
dialogue between service worker and client of a kind that helps to elicit
the client's needs as a self and to determine how they may be best met.
In such dialogue, both worker and client work together to enable the
client's articulation of his or her needs; the worker holds the space
within which the client can learn to trust that it is possible to find his
or her needs through being invited to articulate them and to have
them listened to; the client in learning s/he can trust the relationship
and learn how to work with the service worker has to give of him or
herself in entering and using this relationship. It becomes a mutually
enriching and nourishing relationship.

The contemporary politics of public welfare provision

In the constitutional democracies associated with welfare state formation,
the state has assumed responsibility for governing the welfare services.
Government responsibility for welfare service provision does not mean
that the state is the sole or even primary funding agency for these

services. It does mean, however, that it is the state that determines the policy settings for welfare service provision and, also, what combination of public and private funding commitment prevails, just as it is also the state that guides and directs the network of public, voluntary (not-for-profit), and for-profit agencies that are involved in the delivery of formal welfare services.

As with all institutions, welfare services have to be built over time. Continuous development that permits ongoing learning from experience is of importance to their institutional integrity. So too is the integration of what is happening in the institutional development of welfare services with the training and education of the professionals and paraprofessionals who are the workers who 'deliver' welfare. For a long time in the course of the development of welfare services in the twentieth century such continuous development and its integration with professional education and training seemed relatively secure. The welfare systems were essentially delegated by the state to the professionals who ran the government departments responsible for these different areas who in turn tended to delegate responsibility for direct service provision to the professionals running service agencies. The professional-bureaucratic government of these policy areas matched the responsibility of each profession for regulating itself within a relationship of accountability to public law and norms.

Sometime in the last couple of decades of the twentieth century, this type of public management of welfare services was abandoned by the state which, instead, adopted a highly interventionist, bureaucratic mode of micro-management of them in the name of better or improved performance. The state rhetorically invoked the figure of the service consumer as the *raison d'être* of such reform, and, in so doing, the state espoused the idea of the individual as will. This was also a time that favoured a populist conception of democratic government as one that directly expresses the will of the people, and this easily flowed into an idea that the services the state provides should directly correspond to the will of those who use them. It was also a time that assimilated feminist demands for 'equality' for women in relation to men by extending to women the status of will, thereby creating a universal conception of social adulthood in terms of will. Thus, in order to 'empower' citizens in relation to service delivery, the state redesigned its relationship to service delivery. Instead of an arms-length relationship to it, where the state assumed that professionals responsible for service delivery could be trusted to get on with it under the eye of the government department responsible for ensuring proper use of funds and compliance with policy objectives, the state entered the world of service delivery with the aim of making it perform better on behalf of service clients (see Cooper and Lousada 2005, especially Chapter 3). The subjection of welfare services to performance management has profoundly changed the inner world of service delivery—it is no longer a space of its own that provides protection for service agencies, workers, clients, and client advocates working together to build service delivery that works for all of these differently positioned players. In micro-managing the service delivery relationship, government has stepped way beyond its competence, and, per forcedly, has had to substitute formal performance measures for a more substantive evaluation of front-line service provision that is informed by the different perspectives of the service managers, professionals, individual clients, and client advocate groups. Such direct governmental interference with front-line service provision has also made it much more subject to the ideological preferences of the government of the day.

This has created a situation where the elected government has no compunction about radically discontinuous changes in welfare service policy including abrupt cancellation of existing service types or cut-backs that make it impossible for existing services to be sustained. Let me offer a Canadian example of the latter kind of radical intervention by government with established welfare services that have grown a pro-fessional knowledge base.[5] This example concerns government cuts in counselling positions in an agency dedicated to working with the sur-vivors of childhood sexual abuse.[6] First two young teenage women sur-vivors were interviewed, one having been sexually abused by her brother, the other sexually abused by her father; they spoke of how crucial their access to individual counsellors trained to work in this area has been, and one of them says she would have killed herself if this service had not been available. Both girls emphasized that because of their experience of sexual abuse by family members, trust is a major issue for each of them, and that it has been important for them, as individuals, to have had the opportunity to build and sustain a rela-tionship with an individual counsellor who has got to know their history and with whom they were able to establish trust. They were horrified to learn of the agency's action in laying-off some of the coun-selling staff. This part of the segment concluded with one girl saying to the interviewer 'thanks for listening, so glad to have a voice', with the other girl chiming in with a soft affirmative 'yeah!'

Geraldine Crisci, a specialist in the assessment and treatment of child sexual abuse, who has developed protocols for trauma assessment, and the assessment of sexualized behaviour in children, and who also provides clinical consultation to a variety of sexual abuse treatment programs, children's mental health centres and treatment residences, was also interviewed. In interview, she affirmed the importance of a young person who has experienced child sexual abuse being assessed, and then getting access to the support they need, as soon after the disclosure of the abuse as possible. On the basis of 30 years' experience in the field, she proposed that the single most important fact in recovery is what is done immediately after disclosure; by coming in when the child discloses, she said, we are preventing countless mental health issues for the future. Crisci said funding is always an issue, that when we started this work 30 years ago, we had a lot of funding and we did not know what we were doing at all. Here we are 30 years later and we know a lot, and we are having funding cut, left, right and centre. Crisci said of adult survivors of childhood sexual abuse, who were not fortunate enough to have had access to such services when they were children or young people, they may function, but their quality of life is seriously and negatively affected by severe depression and anxiety. The girl, whose brother sexually abused her, had already spoken of her father as an adult survivor of sexual abuse, and in this small glimpse into the complexity of a family's history, we glimpse something of the intergenerational patterning of the experience of sexual abuse.

Our contemporary welfare debate is essentially not about resources and their allocation, or rather when it is, this is proxy for another debate, one that is conducted within the terrain of subjective attachment to two distinct and opposed ideas of the individual. Where one sees individuality in terms of a self-sufficient will, the other sees individuality in terms of relational possibilities that depend for their outcome on the quality of the inter-subjective engagement between selves.

In the theoretical first part of this book I elaborate on the nature of this debate from the standpoint of articulating the idea of the individual as a self. In the next chapter, I suggest that the idea of the self as the subject of welfare emerged in the twentieth century and that it shaped the evolution of the welfare state in that century. In Chapter 3, I discuss how a societal orientation to knowledge of subjective life has developed an idea of the self that permits the older idea of self-preservation to assume a substance it could not otherwise have. In Chapter 4, I explicitly address the conception of the self as the subject of welfare; while in Chapter 5, I address the contrary conception of individualization—the idea of the will as the subject of welfare. In Chapter 6, I show how the idea of the self as the subject of welfare opens up a conception of the service delivery relationship as inter-subjective process. In Chapter 7, I offer a brief discussion of the impli-cations of individualization understood in terms of the idea of the self for governing welfare services.

In Part II of this book, we turn to the case studies we constructed of welfare services that are oriented to the subject of welfare considered as a self. These case studies are not intended to exhaust possibilities or to be more than they are—historically situated developments that share the limits of their time and place. Nevertheless they represent a rela-tively coherent set of achievements in social policy on the part of the Australian state that deserve to have their story told. They also deserve to be theorized which is what I have sought to do in this first part of the book.

Notes

1 In my 'Varieties of Individualism' (2007a, 49) I propose that 'individualism is a way of thinking about and organizing social life so that it is open to the presence of human social actors as individuals. Whatever it means exactly to enjoy the status of being present as an individual in one's social relations, the essential thing is that the social actor is accorded the standing of one who is legitimately a centre of initiative in these relationships'.

2 Property right, for Locke, is legitimate only as it serves the right to self-preservation; thus he places an ethical limitation on how much property an individual is entitled to (see Tully 1980, Chapter 5, and Tully 1993, Chapter 2).

3 John Locke wrestled with the difficulty of reconciling a universal right of each human being as a person to the right of self-preservation with the private government of the will over the household. He emphatically declared that the master of the household did not have the power of life and death over his wife, children or employees, a right associated with ancient Roman patriarchal power (see Locke 1970, section 86, p. 323). Moreover, Locke based the right of the parents to command the obedience of their children in the obligation of the former to educate their children. He made consent the basis of marriage and the employment relationship; but once inside these relationships, in order to secure the authority of the will, Locke positions the wife and the employee under the government of the master's will. The idea of the will does not preclude the possibility that several individuals can combine to form a joint will or partnership; and Locke assumes this to be true with regard to husband and wife in their parenting role (see for example Locke 1970, section 64, p. 310).

4 I was the reviewer evaluating South Australian Domiciliary Care Services which came under the national Home and Community Care Program. See Yeatman (1989).

5 These would be provincial government cuts. In the early 1990s the Canadian federal government radically devolved responsibility for welfare services to

the provinces in what was already a highly regionalized as distinct from a centralized federal system. Such devolution has had the effect of making the contemporary politics of welfare service provision relatively invisible in national debate.

6   The radio show was broadcast on Radio One by the CBC, May 30 2007; it is called 'The Current' and the interviewer is Anna Maria Tremonti, and I am reporting my notes on my listening to the show. I have taken information about Geraldine Crisci from her Toronto-based consulting firm's website, 'Crisci & Mayer—Consultation, Counseling, Training'.

2
The Twentieth Century Idea of the Self and Its Expression in the Ethos of the Welfare State

The conception of the welfare subject as a self is a twentieth century one. The welfare state, thought of as the public provision of services that make it possible for individuals to enjoy the status of the person, could not have been developed without this idea of the person as a self. Psychoanalysis and psychoanalytically informed ways of thinking placed on the historical agenda the conception of mind as subjective life and a conception of the self understood as a unique centre of subjective life. These ways of thinking exemplified a broader phenomenological movement in thought (see Varela, Thompson and Rosch 1993). The older ethical idea of a right to self-preservation acquired something that had been missing until now: an account of the subject as an embodied self. In this framework, welfare services are services that are designed to facilitate and secure the integrity of the individual considered as a unique centre of subjective-somatic experience.

Here I suggest more continuity than is usually offered in contemporary accounts of the impact of individualization on welfare. Most of these accounts pick the story up in the last quarter of the twentieth century referring especially to social movement advocacy on behalf of the 'active welfare subject' in context of a critique of a top-down and paternalistic type of expert-bureaucratic regime of welfare administration (see Williams 1999; Williams 2000; Harris 1999): 'What began to emerge were new contesting discourses of welfare which ... focused upon the reconstitution of the welfare subject as an active element in the social relations of welfare, rather than the passive recipient of (benevolent or controlling) welfare (Williams 1999, 669)'.

Such accounts are correct so far as they refer to the self-understanding of welfare movement advocacy of this time (for example the women's health movement, the various disability movements, and welfare rights organizations) but they are too partial in their view point, too close to these movements, and too incurious as to the historical conditions that shaped these movements' substantive conception of welfare. Their rejection of a paternalistic style of professionalism should be understood more as a revision than as a rejection of the ethics of professionalism. However, in stressing the agency of the welfare subject, these movements extract the welfare subject from the relationship in which s/he is always to be found: a relationship between the welfare subject and the welfare deliverer. In this respect, there is a discursive consensus shared across these movements' advocacy of welfare user rights and empowerment, on the one hand, and the neo-liberal championship of the welfare subject as a sovereign consumer[1]: the idea of individuality as will. In the one-sided and de-contextualized emphasis on the agency of the welfare subject, there is an inevitable tendency, intended or not, to place professional delivery of the welfare service as means in relation to the ends (choice) that express the will of the welfare subject. This not only takes us up a blind alley—the ethics of welfare cannot be considered just in relation to one term of the relationship—it also obscures the role of welfare professionals in developing the conception of their work as one of facilitation of the integrity of the individual thought of as a unique centre of subjective-somatic experience. It is precisely because the professional does and must have the power to shape the relationship between service deliverer and welfare subject that it is of consequence how the professional thinks of this relationship. If the relationship is to be generative in relation to the integrity of the welfare subject's self and his or her possibilities for growth as a self, then how the professional thinks and acts in such a way as to facilitate this is of vital importance.

Once we include the critical role of professionals in forming the conception of the welfare subject as a unique centre of somatic-subjective experience, we can see that the historical evolution of this idea of welfare services was more continuous over the course of the twentieth century than we would expect if our stress is simply on how the participatory democratic ethos of the new social movements finds its way in to the welfare debates of the 1970s and 1980s. Until the last two decades of the century, those who administered state welfare policy were usually professionals trained in that area who understood how to delegate authority to fellow professionals working in direct service delivery.

In claiming the importance of the role of professional advocacy of this conception of welfare, I am not arguing that all professionals within a particular welfare discipline (medicine, social work, nursing, psychiatry, e.g.) subscribed to it or that even the prevailing view of the profession at a particular time favoured such advocacy. For example Winnicott, a medical doctor and psychoanalyst opposed the psychiatric profession's use of shock treatment and leucotomies in the 1940s and 1950s, methods of treatment that position the patient as a thing rather than as a centre of subjective life.[2] Professionals, no doubt, divide into those who are willing to manage the behaviour of the clients on behalf of goals that are extrinsic to what is of subjective significance to the client, and those who are willing to shape what they have to offer in relation to what is of subjective significance to the client. My argument turns on those professionals who answered the call of the ethical challenge of their times and, in heeding it, responded with a creative account of how best to think about and practically facilitate the well-being of the human subject considered as a self.

Professional vision and advocacy of welfare services in their substantive particularity does not develop independently of what it is that professionals learn from service clients or users both individually and as organized groups. Learning and development in this area of human life is profoundly relational for the core of welfare service work is the relationship between the service deliverer and the service client.

The voices of self-advocates as clients and of the survivors of various kinds of 'systems abuse' (see Cashmore, Dolby and Brennan 1994) in offering their own stories have been of vital importance in the evolution of the conception of the welfare subject as a self. They have contributed to the discrediting of institutional forms of warehousing people, and of other kinds of provider-centred care. Professionals, too, have contributed their own expert evaluation of the damage done to individuals by such practices to public debate, thus feeding the survivor voice with further evidence concerning the injuries and wrongs suffered. In a remarkable book by one of this project's collaborators, Joanna Penglase's account of growing up as a child in institutional care in the period after the Second World War in Australia, we catch a suggestive glimpse of how this collaborative relationship between welfare professionals and clients can work. Here is how she begins the foreword, 'My Story,' to her book:

> For as long as I can remember, I have woken up every morning with a feeling of dread. For me, the story that could not be told was the story of my early loss—the story behind my dread. I could not tell anyone what happened to me because I did not know. Only my analyst could tell, on my behalf, the story that made sense of my life,

of my symptoms, but until I met her there was nobody who was able to do that. That dread has only recently left me. It was exorcised by ten years of therapy which gave me a 'meaningful way' of telling my story for myself (Penglase 2005, 9).

The emergence of the idea of the subject as a whole person—as an embodied self

The subjective experience of the individual considered as unique embodied subject or self gathers increasing attention over the course of the twentieth century. This is someone whose organic life is profoundly affected and mediated by her subjective experience and vice versa. Once conceived as someone whose subjective and organic existence imbricate each other, and in such a way that her being is distinctly her own, the idea of the subject as a 'whole person' can be elaborated.

Here I offer some examples of the idea of the subject as a whole person, as an embodied self, with reference to some key thinker-practitioners whose ability to formulate the idea entered into the practice they led. In offering these examples my intention is to be suggestive rather than to be inclusive; there would be different ways of telling a similar story. The key figures I select straddle a time that connects the nineteenth century world of their intellectual and actual parents and the participatory movements of the late twentieth century.

Psychoanalysis is central to the development of the idea of the subject as a whole person or embodied self. Donald Winnicott (1897–1971) is a leading figure who offered insight into the integration of somatic and psychic aspects of the subject's existence as a self. In 1949, Winnicott proposed that 'the word psyche ... means the imaginative elaboration of somatic parts, feelings, and functions, that is, of physical aliveness (Winnicott 1992b, 244)'. Here Winnicott was elaborating an insight that Melanie Klein (1882–1960) and her followers had contributed to psychoanalytic thought: that the individual's experience of his or her organic drives is always mediated by phantasy: 'there is no impulse, no instinctual urge or response which is not experienced as unconscious phantasy (Isaacs, 1989, 83)'.

Moshe Feldenkrais (1904–1984), a contemporary of Winnicott, developed a method of somatic education that is predicated also on the centrality of somatic experience to subjective experience. Feldenkrais's insights, belonging as they did to a particular *zeitgeist* (see Yeatman 2007c), have turned out to anticipate the new sciences of mind (Varela, Thompson and Rosch 1993; Siegel 1999; Siegel 2007; Fonagy *et al.* 2004).

For Feldenkrais, movement is the most accessible and functionally significant expression of the quality of aliveness each of us as an individual subject experiences. He suggests the complexity of the psyche- soma relationship when he proposes that, for reasons of our upbringing and emotional experience, aspects of our embodiment remain outside our somatic experience—they remain latent and unarticulated. They do not enter our 'self-image', as he calls it, which means we do not draw upon these parts of our embodied self in order to function—to move which includes, of course, our capacity to breathe. The quality of our functioning depends on how much of our self we engage in our functioning. If our self image is partial rather than complete, our potential for movement will be restricted in ways that compromise our sense of being alive in a pleasurable and creative way (see the chapter on 'the self image' in Feldenkrais 1990). The entire orientation of the Feldenkrais method of teaching and learning is to facilitate the opening of new ways of using our selves so as to fill out our self image. This is done through a teacher's facilitation of the growth of the individual's capacity to become aware of how she senses herself in movement. If the individual's range of capacity expands, then the individual is freer to do what s/he may want to do. 'How can I know what I want if I do not know how I do?' is a question that Moshe Feldenkrais asks in his 'Awareness through Movement' lessons as we access them today (in recordings and transcripts). In his chapter on self-image, Feldenkrais (1990, 19) makes it clear that improvement of self-image presupposes that we have learnt to value ourselves as individuals rather than as members of the group: 'It is important to understand that if a man wishes to improve his self-image, he must first learn to value himself as an individual'. In expanding her somatic awareness, the individual becomes a more resilient self, knowing that she is able to find a way of unlocking herself when, as is inevitable, she retreats into familiar but deeply compromised patterns of self use.

Feldenkrais scorned psychoanalysis but what he was doing for the facilitation of individual self experience in a somatic sense, psychoanalysis and the psychoanalytically-influenced currents of psychotherapy were doing for the facilitation of individual self experience in a psychic sense. Both methods are oriented to the development of a self awareness that enable a more alive and more integrated way of being an embodied self. Both methods are predicated on the proposition that the psychoanalyst Thomas Ogden (1996, 19) takes from Freud: 'there is only one mental life comprised of the product of (dynamically) unconscious and conscious psychical qualities'. Thinking as self-awareness is a lighting up of our being in a way that invites new patterns of self-regulation, and such thinking is only partially conveyed in words for it is a dynamic activity on the part of the whole self.

While psychoanalysis may seem to have been an esoteric practice in relation to the mainstream of welfare state services as they developed in the twentieth century, this is not so. In Britain the Tavistock Institute has been an extraordinarily important point of intersection between psychoanalytic thought and welfare service practice, especially but not only in social work. The relationship of psychoanalysis to medicine is worth considering. There is something of a shared ethos between psychoanalysis and late nineteenth century and twentieth century medicine up until about the last three decades of the twentieth century. Donald Winnicott was trained as a medical doctor from 1917–1920 (see Rodman 2003, 38), and Clare Winnicott, his wife, says of his training: 'Donald had some great teachers at the hospital, and he always said that it was Lord Horder who taught him the importance of taking a careful case history, and to listen to what the patient said, rather than simply to ask questions (C. Winnicott 1989, 12)'.[3] She (1989, 13) says also that he 'had always intended to become a general practitioner in a country area, but one day a friend lent him a book by Freud, and so he discovered psychoanalysis'.

It is not surprising that Winnicott was attracted to general practice medicine for this was a time when general practice involved a generalist training in all core medical competences (surgery, diagnosis, pharmacology) and was oriented to the treatment of the patient as a whole person. I know of this ethos first hand from my father John Yeatman (1914–2006) whose father and grandfather were also general practitioners working in South Australia. My father's medical hero was the Canadian physician, William Osler (1849–1919), whose 'greatest contribution to medicine was to insist that students learned from seeing and talking to patients and the establishment of the medical residency program' rather than have them just sit in a lecture hall, taking notes. The Wikipedia entry (on which I am drawing for this information about Osler) continues:

> He himself liked to say, 'He who studies medicine without books sails an uncharted sea, but he who studies medicine without patients does not go to sea at all'. He is also remembered for saying, 'If you listen carefully to the patient they will tell you the diagnosis'.

A further Osler quote from the same source: 'It is much more important to know what sort of a patient has a disease than what sort of a disease a patient has'. My father's way of putting this was to say that the patient is always her own best doctor. Osler also offered a conception of medicine as a 'science of uncertainty and an art of probability'.

There would have been few general practitioners, working as they did until fairly recently with the same individual patients and their children over the course of their respective life histories, who did not intuit the complexity of the relationship between somatic and psychic aspects of self experience and who did not develop insight into the socially contextual aspects of individual health and illness. Robertson Davies, the Canadian novelist, distils something of the ethos of early and mid-twentieth century general practice medicine in the reflections of the doctor who is the central character in *The Cunning Man*:

> Because I was not devising a new notion of medicine; I was seeking a very old one, a sort of perennial philosophy of the healer's art, and fatality, or necessity, was the element in life that kept me humble, for nothing I could ever do would defeat it. People must be ill, and they must die. If I could seem to postpone the dark day people thought me a good doctor, but I knew it was a postponement, never a victory, and I could secure a postponement only if Fatality, the decision of my patient's *daimon*, so directed.

> Of course I could not say that sort of thing to the anxious patient sitting in the chair opposite me. (I never sit behind a desk; always in a chair opposite to the patient and no greater in importance than his.) Who wants to hear his doctor saying that he must die sometime, and the doctor cannot say when, and that anything that can be done in the meantime will not change that fact? And in virtually all cases something could be done, some physical comfort assured, some assuagement of pain or disability, until the inevitable happened.

> ... I was not a convinced believer in anything the enthusiasts for psychosomatic medicine have to say, though I was an intent listener. Of course the mind influences the body; but the body influences the mind, as well, and to take only one side in the argument is to miss much that is—in the true sense of the word—vital. Didn't Montaigne say, with that splendid wisdom that was so much his own, that the close stitching of mind to body meant that

each communicated its fortunes to the other? (Davies 1995, 330–331).

Medicine in its largely intuitive sense of the mutual imbrication of somatic and psychic life went only so far for it remained insistently a bio-medical science so that the interpretive art of working with subjective experience took a back seat. It was psychoanalysis that was responsible for the rich knowledge of subjective life that developed over the course of the twentieth century, especially the psychoanalysis focused on the development of the infant after birth. Melanie Klein made it possible to view the infant as already a centre of subjective experience. In the wake of her ideas, and buttressed by the empirical contribution of infant observation that became part of Kleinian-influenced psychoanalytic training, came the work of Esther Bick, Wilfred Bion and Frances Tustin (see Mitrani 2001, Chapter 2; as well as Briggs 2002). They could presuppose also Winnicott's contribution of the idea of 'the facilitating environment' and Bowlby's work on attachment theory, which together with Bion's idea of containment, offered the core insight that the baby cannot achieve unit status (Winnicott's term) as a self-organized unit of being unless it has the good fortune to experience a form of holding itself (and thus its experience) together from how her parent(s) care for and interact with him or her.

Esther Bick (1901–1983), who developed the method of infant observation, disagreed with Melanie Klein's proposition that the infant has an ego at birth, and proposed instead that the baby's being is 'in pieces' until it is able to bind the parts of itself together through contact with its maternal object (Briggs 2002, 8–9). Bick thus agreed with Winnicott that it is the mother who in the first instance holds the baby's parts together—passively from the standpoint of the baby (see Briggs 2002, 7–14). Bion's (1994) conception of how the parent/analyst provides containment for the baby's/patient's intolerable experiences so that it becomes possible for this subject to bear these feelings and thus to 'have' its experience rather than to fragment its experience by flinging it away or projecting it onto someone else, is a similar idea. It is only if the baby can have its experience that it can embark on the process of self-integration.

The construction of the subject as an individual unit of embodied mind was significant not just for the idea it offered of the individual as a whole person whose existence would be all the more functional if the individual could function in his or her wholeness, that is, enable all his or her aspects of self to become developed, and, thus, to be available to him or her as s/he needs them. It also made it clear that the conception of individuality in terms of will—the disciplines of self-mastery and self-improvement—is a costly and dysfunctional form of self use because it makes it impossible to practice aliveness in an integrated way. The use of will to master the self encourages the individual to split off those aspects of self that are not amenable to being mastered. Such splitting is destructive of the integrity of the individual and of the possibilities of growth as a self. This is an alternative way of thinking about the self as one who is able to integrate awareness of both the good and bad aspects of its being and who is able to tolerate internal conflict. For Winnicott (and for the Kleinian current of psychoanalytic thought generally) this is the measure of psychic health. As Winnicott puts it in his talk on 'The meaning of the word "democracy"':

> ... the healthy person, who is capable of being depressed, is able to find the whole conflict within the self as well as able to see the whole conflict outside the self, in external (shared) reality. When healthy persons come together, they each contribute a whole world, because each brings a whole person (Winnicott 1986, 244).

In shifting from the will to the self, it was possible also to abandon the notion that the self has to assume a coherence that is expressible in a rational mode of wording a preference. Once the internal complexity of the self could be acknowledged, self-awareness is simply a way of lighting up or disclosing self experience as it is framed by the question that the self asks of itself. Such questions change all the time in relation to different kinds of activity, relationship, and shifting contextual circumstance, so that what the self reflexively knows today has an evanescent quality even though it informs current preferences and the dynamic process by which a person comes to achieve a capacity for self knowledge.

The acknowledgment of subjective experience in the ethos of the welfare state

To my knowledge there has not been much work done on the ethos that informed the development of the welfare state. There is the established view that the welfare state was a vehicle for the development of citizenship status, but there has not been much enquiry into the conception of the citizen as a subject of need for welfare services. My contention is that the idea of the individual as an embodied subject, and as a centre of subjective experience, as developed in medicine, psycho-analysis, and other disciplines, underpins this idea of the citizen as a subject of need. As we have seen, post-Freudian psychoanalysis empha-sizes the coming into being of a self in context of attachment to others which can be more or less functional. Both psychoanalysis and the Feldenkrais method assume that self-integration has to be facilitated by another subject. Thus, the idea of individuality they offer is one that views the self as an ecology of relationships, both internal and external to the self. In social work the idea of the self as an ecology of attach-ments was articulated in an emphasis on 'the individual in his family and social setting' (Woodroofe 1962, 211).[4]

The older idea of self-preservation is oriented to the valuing of each human being as a subject, and as I propose in the next chapter, it is this idea of subjective right that is at the core of human rights. The development of a welfare service ethos of responsiveness to the indi-vidual as a self presupposes the valuing of the individual as the subject of right. In this respect, the ethos of welfare can be viewed as an elabo-ration of the idea of a right to self preservation. The twentieth century development of 'social security' should not be seen independently of this history for why should people have their 'social security' attended to as a matter of public policy unless it is the case that their status as selves who deserve to be preserved has become a matter of public value?

Prior to the twentieth century the provision for the welfare of those who needed support and assistance was governed by the ethos of the patriarchal household economy whether this was expressed at the level of the family household, a charitable institution, or of the state. There were thus three possibilities of provision for need. The first of these was dependence on private familial and/or extended familial support, for example, the nursing at home of an elderly parent, or the adoption of an orphaned child by relatives; the second of these was dependence on private charitable institutions such as asylums; the third was depen-dence on a government-regulated system of public relief which in Britain after 1834 involved the institutional order of a 'general mixed workhouse system' (Hirst and Michael 2003, 147).[5] The system of public relief was designed to make employment rather than relief the preferable option for people who were deemed able to work. Public relief was a system of control of the poor where it was assumed that if they could be made to serve societal ends by gainful employment, this would serve also their own individual ends (see de Schweinitz 1961, Chapters 3, 5 and 6). It is fair to say that the objective underlying the containment of different kinds of need, distress and abjection was one of protection of the group rather than the individual. There was nothing in such provision for need that secured the status of the individual as the subject of right; on the contrary—to be subject to those who provided for need was a form of slavery in the sense of subjection to the arbitrary will of others.

The trajectory for welfare services for most of the twentieth century was to provide a base of income and service support for people who needed them in such a way as to respect their status as an individual subject of right, as a person. In the twentieth century welfare provision came to be regarded as a question of entitlement such as to permit the individual to maintain his or her dignity and sense of self.

The valuing of the individual as the subject of need owes much to the increased understanding of subjective life. While thinkers like those I have mentioned in the preceding section formulated this understanding, it had to have a corresponding presence in everyday historical experience. One major historical opening for the development of such an everyday understanding of subjective experience occurred through the First World War and the phenomenon of 'shell-shock'. 'According to one estimate, mental breakdowns represented 40 per cent of British casualties' (Herman 2001, 20). Judith Herman's account of the medical response to such breakdowns is instructive. It suggests something of the processes by which inner life or subjective experience of the individual began to acquire currency. Of course these processes had precursors (e.g. in the nineteenth century romantic movement's exploration of subjective experience) and they did not occur all at once. They unfolded in fits and starts, and they were always contested.

Herman (2001, 20–21) proposes that once 'the existence of a combat neurosis could no longer be denied, medical controversy ... centred on the moral character of the patient'. In the traditionalist view, as she calls it, 'a normal soldier should glory in war and betray no sign of emotion'. A soldier who was subjectively traumatized by war 'was at best a constitutionally inferior human being, at worst a malingerer and a coward (Herman 2001, 21)'. This is a view of the soldier not unlike the idea of the able-bodied individual who depends on welfare relief as a malingerer, 'dole bludger', and someone who is willing to take taxpayers' contributions to the public purse without assuming his fair share of responsibility. Herman mentions Lewis Yealland, a British psychiatrist, who 'advocated a treatment strategy based on shaming, threats, and punishment', similar to the reinvention of the 1834 British Poor

Law in contemporary 'workfare' approaches to people dependent on public income support. Herman (2001, 21) suggests violent means of disciplining the lazy and cowardly soldier were advocated by Yealland: 'Hysterical symptoms such as mutism, sensory loss, or motor paralysis were treated with electric shocks'. This punitive approach presupposed that the malingering will had to be broken if the moral will was to be restored. This approach not only failed but it was challenged by W.H.R. Rivers who accepted that the symptoms presented by the soldiers were *bona fide*. Herman (2001, 22) discusses Rivers's alternative treatment of Siegfried Sassoon, a poet who became a pacifist through his experience in the war:

> The goal of all treatment, as in all military medicine, was to return the patient to combat. Rivers did not question this goal. He did, however, argue for the efficacy of a form of talking cure. Rather than being shamed, Sassoon was treated with dignity and respect. Rather than being silenced, he was encouraged to write and talk freely about the terrors of war.

The shift here was important: subjective difficulty of a kind that means the individual concerned is unable to function in socially expected ways was no longer understood as expressive of lack of moral character, but as making sense in terms of the subjective experience of the individual in trying to cope with an extraordinarily challenging and traumatic environment. Since World War I the idea of the subjective impact of trauma has become increasingly current. Beverley Raphael (2005, 31) comments of the idea of trauma as it is now used:

> Psychological trauma has become the lens through which all adversity is viewed. ... At the end of this spectrum of response is the diagnosis of post traumatic stress disorder—recognized in earlier times by many different names including Freud's concept of 'traumatic neurosis', 'shell-shock' after World War I and 'combat fatigue' after World War II. ... Trauma in the psychological sense has, of course, been recognised well beyond the wounds of war. It has appeared with the violence of the home: domestic violence and child abuse—the battered wife and the battered child syndromes in the earlier stages; and, of course, the victims of disaster and more recently terrorism.

World War II also provided a laboratory of sorts for child psycho-analysts like Winnicott and Bowlby who studied the psychological effects of the evacuation of children away from their families in London to the countryside on them, as well as other kinds of separation between children and their families (the *Kindertransport* of Jewish children; the use of group nurseries to allow mothers to contribute to the war effort). This provided Bowlby with information he could use for the development of attachment theory. Winnicott, who emphasized the importance of stable, ongoing maternal provision of a 'facilitating environment' for the psychic maturation of babies and children was reputed to have said 'children would have been better off bombed than evacuated'.[6]

After World War II the foundations of what came to be called 'the welfare state' were laid in extensive provision of income support services, access to medical services and educational services. This was also the era of the end of legitimacy for the institutionalization of individuals (children in care, young people in reformatories, people with mental illness, people with cognitive impairment, and older frail people who could not manage to live independently any more). Either community-based alternatives or congregate care designed on a more human scale and in such a way that the needs of people as individuals could be accommodated, were now advocated and led to new service types in the 1970s, 1980s and 1990s.

Once the subjective experience of infants and children began to be acknowledged an entire underbelly of social life began to be exposed. It become increasingly clear towards the end of the twentieth century that children who had been institutionalized had been subject to routine humiliation, neglect and abuse, including sexual abuse, and this new knowledge converged with increasing awareness of intra-familial relationships of domination and abuse. So endemic are these phenomena that it is not possible to blame them on a few 'bad apples' even if it is clear that society in its popular media is still struggling with what it means to acknowledge the ordinariness of these phenomena. Moral character, it is clear, has not stopped many socially upstanding abusers from abusing vulnerable subjects. On this and other fronts, there begins to be a societal curiosity as to how it is that an individual's subjective experience or inner life has become so organized that it leads this individual to abuse others. There is a generalized acceptance that if an individual has him or herself suffered trauma, unless s/he is facilitated in coming to accept these painful and shameful aspects of his or her self experience, s/he is unlikely to be able to contain them as distinct from acting them out.

There is also currently a generalized acceptance that poverty in an affluent society, where accordingly the social division between those who are poor and those who are affluent is marked in status terms, has a subjective impact. Harry Ferguson (2003, 207–209) sustains this way of thinking when he speaks of poor people under sustained inner and external stress, who do not have enough material resources to relax into parenting, who have/had child abuse/care problems in relation to their own children, and had experienced abuse in their own childhood. He (2003, 209) proposes: 'a central issue in theorising reflexivity [what I have been calling self awareness] and the (excluded) welfare subject concerns the intersection of structural disadvantage and personal biography and how people adjust to adversity and cope with toxic experiences and relationships in their lives'. Paul Hoggett (2008, 80) speaks of 'the rage, the pain and the despair which welfare professionals work with on a daily basis'. He refers to and quotes a youth worker with over 20 years experience who ran 'a remarkably successful youth club on a housing estate which has long had a notorious reputation':

> He's referring to a recent incident in which some youths trashed his club and then three of them—two brothers and their friend's cousin—turned on each other. The younger brother is known to be dangerous and has used knives in the past.

> The younger brother and the other protagonist were just yelling abuse at each other. And they sounded so hysterical, fragile and upset. I mean that was quite upsetting, because they were both saying really hurtful things to each other. I mean when I find this, all of them have actually got quite a lot of pain in their backgrounds and they scratch at each other's pain, they don't let it, they don't show solidarity for other people. On these situations they pull at the scabs you know, yelling awful things about their parents, the majority of which were true, you know (Hoggett 2008, 80).

The particular value of Hoggett's work (Hoggett 2000; 2001; 2008) is that he insists not only on the complexities and difficulties in working with individuals whose sense of self has been profoundly damaged but that, as indicated in this example, their behaviour can be such as to evoke for good reasons hatred in the welfare worker. It is important not to idealize the welfare subject; subjective life is not just messy and chaotic but also has dark aspects. In applying it to his own analysis of abused women who as mothers have got caught up in the child protection system, Ferguson (2003, 212) usefully summarizes this aspect of Hoggett's work thus:

> Hoggett identifies three subject positions in welfare: victim, own worst enemy, and creative, reflexive agent. What the present analysis shows is the complex reality that very often the most needy clients of services can occupy two or all of these positions at once.

Once infants, a category of subject that obviously cannot govern itself, could be conceptualized as already existent in an emotional/psychic sense, it became possible to rethink the subjective existence of all people who suffered some kind of mental impairment. As Valerie Sinason (1992) put it, if the mind itself is alive (and it may not be), then there will be emotional intelligence in the most mentally impaired individual. On this basis the idea of warehousing people in institutions, where they were subject to being managed in batches, often abused, and kept quiet, could become seen as the horror it is.

If it became possible to conceive the individual as a self who suffers the vicissitudes of life, it became also possible to work with the subjective aspects of death and dying. The idea of palliative care and advocacy of euthanasia were central to the development of the hospice movement in the 1960s and 1970s (Maddocks 2005, 54). Support for the individual in how s/he wants to die was also provoked by the HIV-AIDs epidemic in the 1980s at the time when there was no cure. Pat Jalland (2005, 14) suggests there has been a growing acceptance of death and dying as central to the existential experience of the human condition, a shift from a more stoic culture to one that welcomes more open expressions of grief, and a reaction against the over-medicalisation of death in hospitals.

Conclusion

In this chapter I have historically charted in a suggestive rather than systemic way the ways in which the individual thought of as a centre of embodied mind—as a centre of subjective experience—came to assume currency in the twentieth century. I have argued that it is this idea of the individual, accompanied by the proposition that the individual's right to self preservation should be secured, that informed the normative vision for the twentieth century welfare state. My intention has been one of seeking to historically situate the idea of the subject of welfare considered as self, to suggest it did not come out of nowhere, but belongs to an entire and complex history. In the next chapter I elaborate on the idea of the individual as a centre of subjective experience in relation to the idea of subjective right or the right to self-preservation.

Notes

1   Fiona Williams (1999, 669) emphasizes this aspect of consensus: 'The challenges to the so-called consensus supporting the post-war Keynesian welfare settlement came thick and fast in a variety of forms: economic recession, the 'unfixing' of gender and ethnic relations, changes in the organization and provision of employment, demographic shifts, challenges to the sovereignty of the nation-state. They fed into political challenges to the welfare state which emerged during the 1970s and which focused upon the nature of its key organizational characteristics—mass/universal, state provided, bureaucratically run and professionally-delivered. The challenges came from both neoliberal critiques of the welfare state's efficiency and from progressive critiques of its universality and accountability developed from the new forms of political collectivities on the left—originally from the social movements based in inequalities of gender, race, disability and sexuality, but later also from groups organized around specific welfare rights and needs'.

2   Winnicott's opposition is expressed in writings reproduced in Part Four of Winnicott (1989a). In one of these writings, a letter to the editor of the *British Medical Journal*, he says: 'Actually I do not see how permission is ever obtained for the treatment to be done, as there is good evidence that when an adult gives permission for it to be done on himself he does it out of an impulse which is akin to a suicidal one. What makes a man like hurting himself makes him feel like allowing and even asking for shock treatment. The ethics of collaboration with this suicidal impulse is doubtful'. He says further: 'There is such a thing as a doctor's unconscious antagonism to ill people who do not respond to his therapy. In my opinion shock therapy is too violent a treatment for us to be able to make use of it, at the same time being sure that we are not unconsciously intending it to hurt the patient (Winnicott 1989, 522)'.

3   Rodman (2003, 38) elaborates in his biography of Winnicott: 'The emphasis [in 1918] that Dr Thomas Horder (later Lord Horder) placed on listening carefully to the patient was apparently not a common one. Donald would one day say that psychoanalysis was actually only an extension of this process of history taking'.

4   Woodroofe (1962, 211) cites the British Report on the Working Party of Social Workers in the Local Authority Health and Welfare Services (1959) in this passage: 'The Younghusband Report has recently reminded us ... "There is always a risk in any type of specialization of concentrating on a particular aspect at the expense of the whole", it warns, "... (and) this can lead to a focusing of effort on a particular need or handicap, rather than on the effect of these on the individual in his family or social setting". Accordingly, to do its job properly, a social service must understand the common social and personal factors in the needs of those using the services; it must take into

account needs other than those it was set up to meet, and always the focus must be on the individual in his family and social setting'.

5 'With the spread of the general mixed workhouse system, institutional-isation of pauper "idiots" not cared for by their families became the norm, either in workhouses or, sometimes, the county asylum. By 1861 only 16.2% of recorded "lunatics" and "idiots" in England were outside institutions, and successive records show only continuing confinement in asylum or work-house (Hirst and Michael 2003, 147)'.

6 This was part of remarks given by William Gillespie (cit Rodman 2003, 51) in a memorial tribute to Winnicott in 1972; Gillespie was highlighting Winni-cott's combination of courage, gentleness, and ruthlessness.

3
The Individual as the Centre of Subjective Experience and the Right to Self-preservation

How individualization impacts on the delivery of welfare services depends essentially on the idea of the individual that is in play. I have suggested that there are two distinct ideas of the individual that have quite different implications for how we conceive welfare services and their delivery. The first of these ideas is the individual considered as a unique centre of subjective experience, a self; the second is the individual considered as the subject who wills or chooses—the individual considered as will.

If being an individual is said to involve being a will that is free to choose, then well-being in this conception centres on the freedom to choose, and right concerns the right of the individual to exercise such freedom. So far as this is a public ethic, the role of the state is one of legally demarcating what belongs to whom, thus indicating clear boundaries between the jurisdictional sphere of action of one will relative to another. What goes on within the jurisdictional sphere of action of the will, as long as it is lawful, is of private rather than public concern. All that the individual needs from others is recognition of the lawful exercise of his or her will. Within the jurisdiction of the will is placed such property as the individual owns. In this framework, the norm that individuals seek to realize, and one that the state does what it can to support, is one of individuals possessing sufficient private property to attend to the needs of welfare both of them selves and their familial dependants (children notably, but also other relatives who may come under the family's care). The state's role in matters of welfare provision in this framework is residual; it supplements rather than displaces the private welfare economy of the will.

The alternative idea of the individual as self implicates an entirely different institutional design than that which centres on the will.

Matters are not quite as simple as publicly institutionalizing an arrangement where each individual has the freedom to make private arrangements for attending to his or her welfare and that of his or her dependants. Here the question of individual welfare or well-being concerns the conditions under which the human subject can assume and sustain life as a self. Whether a human being gets to enjoy life as a self does not depend simply on what it is that this individual does or does not do as this is recognized by others. Rather, enjoyment of life as a self depends both on the initiative of the person concerned and on how relevant others positively invite, welcome, facilitate and support this initiative. The welfare of the self, then, concerns a relationship, or set of relationships, between self and other selves. Accordingly, so far as the idea of the self is the basis of a public ethics, the role of the state is one of facilitating and supporting this set of relationships.

When the focus is on the conditions of possibility of a subject assuming life as a self, the availability and quality of parenting of the individual assumes a critical importance. In this frame it is the role of the state to non-intrusively support those who provide parenting to children. It is in the parenting relationship, that the life chances of the subject as a self are constituted. Much now is known of how an internal state of depression can compromise the ability of the mother of a new-born baby to call her baby into live company, thereby joyously welcoming her baby as the self that it is, and tuning her responses to his needs in such a way as to facilitate this baby's articulation of his needs. Anne Alvarez (2002, 68), whose work I particularly draw on here, speaks of 'the mother claiming her baby as her own, claiming his attention, calling him into relation with her and, in a way, calling him into psychological being'. This is a process that involves the mother as one centre of subjective animation (I use this idea of centre of animation from Sheets-Johnstone 1999) calling the other into sharing 'live company' with her. For this to occur the mother has to feel alive, rather than dead as depression causes her to feel. The welfare of the baby as a self coming into being is at risk with a 'dead mother' (Bollas 2001). Depression is a fact of human life, and thus something to be understood and anticipated in the provision of social services. Such anticipation can inform among other things the provision of services that provide both pre- and post-natal support to mothers. Alvarez (2002, 72) comments here:

It should be clear from the evidence and the arguments for an interactional object-relations theory, that the 'cause' of cognitive deficit or emotional withdrawal, or both, in a baby can never be entirely in the mother. The child development research ... has been careful to show that social and cultural supports (a companion, preferably the husband present at the birth, support in the home afterwards, a good marriage, socioeconomic level) all affect whether there is a benign or vicious circle of development. ... Help is often available from skilled health visitors and other types of worker—physiotherapists, child psychotherapists and sometimes helpful nannies, grandmothers and friends—if the situation is treated soon enough. Often, time is on the side of health, and the mother and baby get together in the end. Where not, psychotherapeutic treatment may have to step in where prevention has been lacking.

More generally, if there were more elaborated societal acknowledgment of the vital importance of the quality of parenting to the life chances of the subject as a self, there would be more elaboration of public support for people in their role as parents than there is currently. The idea of the individual as will obstructs such acknowledgment. In the moral economy of the will, there is a simple distinction made between two subject categories: (a) those who instantiate a mature, rational capacity to will/choose for themselves, and, as necessary, for others; and (b) those who lack this capacity for reasons either of developmental immaturity or impairment. Other than the necessity to educate the immature will of the child, there is no attention within this framework to relationship of parenting.

In the framework guided by the idea of the individual as a self, there is also an emphasis on the ongoing challenges for the development of the individual as a self through all his or her different life stages and in relation to different kinds of vicissitude. The self constantly has to undo previous ways of organizing and integrating its being and to learn new ones as it enters new stages of life and faces new external challenges. Psycho-therapeutic, life-counselling, spiritual and other kinds of relationship that facilitate the individual's growth as a self can make the difference to whether an individual is able to bear emotional difficulty, to incorporate it into his or her experience, and to be able to think about it. Where individuals are not supported in such profoundly challenging processes of self-acceptance and self-knowledge, their modes of adaptation to unbearable inner difficulties are likely to be destructive of self, and of others. In this frame of reference, the capacity to think well follows rather than directs the individual's capacity to be open to his or her subjective experience.

Subjective experience is a complex and dynamic set of relationships between the individual's internal world and his or her external worlds. It constitutes the ecology of the individual. It makes sense, then, to think of thinking as a reflexive ordering of subjective experience. If such thinking is to be intelligent, subjective experience has to be available to it; in which case, individuals have to be adequately facilitated and supported in their capacity to face difficult feelings rather than to adopt defences against feelings where such defences must impair both the aliveness of the individual and his or her capacity to think. Without such openness on the part of the individual to his or her subjective experience, it is impossible for him or her to accept and know the suffering of his or her fellows. When s/he adopts inner defences against feeling, such defences must inform what it is s/he can bear to know and accept in the lives of others.

This way of thinking about the individual raises the question whether we can consider an emotionally intelligent social policy (this is a question that Cooper and Lousada 2005, raise in their excellent book on 'feeling and fear of feeling in modern welfare'). This is a question that opens up at a time when the subjective aspect of social life seems to have come onto our collective agenda. If we are now ready to know something of subjective trauma in its ordinary as well as its extraordinary aspects, and to accept how damaging human relationships can be especially to those who for some reason are marked as vulnerable, then perhaps we are ready to engage in public discussion about how best to resource and support front-line welfare professionals who work with the most traumatized people in our society. In their discussion of the Victoria Climbié Report,[1] Cooper and Lousada (2005) propose that good process and procedure in child protection work cannot take the place of in-depth professional supervision that supports child protection workers' emotional capacity to do this appallingly difficult work. They propose:

> There are many cumulative factors in recent years that tend to impede the requirement and the capacity of child protection staff to properly listen to children, and make appropriate relationships with them. ... [There is] a deeper dynamic that is always in play in this kind of work. This is the continual and perfectly understandable wish on the part of workers to believe that what they are being presented with is not a case of child abuse. Because accepting that it is, or that it probably is, pitches them into immediate personal engagement with conflict, emotional pain, and the welter of difficult

feelings and responses [already discussed] ... It is in fact only human not to want to be obliged to enter this territory.

So, time and time again, the evidence of the inquiry report is that workers involved in Victoria's case *both saw and did not see what was in front of their own eyes* ... In ordinary language we call this 'turning a blind eye'. With one part of our mind we take in what is happening, but with another we repudiate what we have seen. This means we are unable to struggle consciously with the conflict, the dilemma, or with the anxiety arising from it; but neither do we make a complete psychological break with the unwelcome knowledge or suspicion of which we are aware, which would be to enter a state of true denial. Rather we disconnect, we break the relationship between different but actually related aspects of, or responses to, a single state of affairs while retaining some kind of consciousness of each. We do this, and it is a very ordinary defences, when we are deeply conflicted about what we are seeing, or about what we have come to know (Cooper and Lousada 2005, 160–161).

Child protection workers cannot do their job well if they are not given support to do this work. It is vitally important that these workers have sustained and ready access to supervision that addresses 'the difficult psychological and emotional transactions that child protection work necessarily involves' (Cooper and Lousada 2005, 162). Yet, as these authors remark, 'it is also the dimension of professional supervision that has been most eroded in the last two decades of child protection work' (Cooper and Lousada 2005, 163).

When the idea of the subject as a self enters into societal discourse, we develop an awareness that the fate and fortune of any one self depends on the relationships that this individual experiences from its birth into the human world. In the elaboration of such awareness, we also begin to realize that if the fortune of the individual depends on its treatment at the hands of others, then how the sense of self of these others has been formed is at issue. Simply put, we are able to understand that how people treat other people is a question of their own subjective history. If they have been subject to violence at the hands of others, such violence will continue to mark their inner life, and cause them to act destructively towards them selves and towards others. Once this kind of understanding of subjective experience has been achieved, we are ready to go beyond a simple moralistic splitting of people into those who are 'good', and those who are 'bad'. We are ready to engage in understanding what kind of subjective experience invites an adult to destroy the subjective and, maybe also, physical integrity of a child in his or her care. Most such destruction is of the ordinary garden variety kind where the adults concerned have capacities for intelligent and generous responses to other selves mixed up with destructive, greedy, envious, and murderous responses to other selves. It takes considerable emotional work to be able to know both these two aspects of oneself or one's parent or another close relative, to hold them in conjunction without wanting to emotionally simplify matters by splitting one aspect off from the other, thus concluding this person is really a bad, or really a good, person.

Societally speaking we are at the beginning of this difficult work, and there is a strange dynamic that operates when we begin to engage in exploration of the vicissitudes of the life of the self in the company of other selves. The very possibility of knowing the dark sides of inter-subjectivity necessarily invites our resistance to such knowledge. So we proceed in half-starts with considerable pressure from various sources, including the media, to collude in moralistic over-simplification, and, thus, to retreat from where we seemed ready to go.

It is no longer adequate to see social policy in terms of provision for the right of each individual to self-preservation where what is at issue is the 'physical' survival of the individual. Now the right to self-preservation begins to be reframed in terms of the coming into being and sustaining for each individual of a sense of self. This conception of the right to self-preservation poses new demands on social policy. It now has to be conceived as a policy environment that facilitates the growth of individuals as selves and where the complexities and difficulties of emotional life are both accepted and brought within the 'unending activity' of understanding (Arendt 1994, 307). Such social policy would assume responsibility for non-intrusively facilitating how people parent their children, and extend also to appropriate facilitation and support of front-line welfare work. It would extend also to support for psycho-therapeutic services that enable young people and adults to come to know and to heal a damaged sense of self. Last but not least social policy so conceived must encourage and facilitate public discussion and conversation of the kind that weaves the fabric of what Hegel called ethical life, a public culture wherein each human subject is invited to be a person who is able to recognize others as persons too.

We might say that the widest set of relationships that inform the conditions of possibility of each individual human being enjoying life as a self are those that belong to the political community that constitutes the public life of the state. The quality of public life is central to the welfare for the self. As Cooper and Lousada (2005, 86) put it, 'the quality of ... welfare rests upon the nature of the shared belief that reciprocity between and obligation towards others is the basis of social concern and citizenship'. It is not just that the citizen says, 'there for the grace of god, go I' in witnessing difficulties in enjoying life as a self on the part of individuals who have suffered trauma, life-threatening illness, unemployment, poverty, and mental illness; but that the citizen has the capacity to think about subjective experience. Here the state's role in providing an integrated and inclusive public culture where all aspects of the human condition are welcomed into public discussion so that they may be known and thought about, and where all those who belong to the political community are honoured as centres of subjective experience, is crucial to the growth of this capacity in the individual citizen. On the other hand, if the state is oriented to an exclusive public culture, one that welcomes those who can attain publicly sanctioned normative standards of behaviour, but moralistically condemns those who cannot or do not, then the individual citizen's capacity to think about subjective experience will be undermined by this splitting of the human condition into what is deemed good and what is deemed bad, with the accompanying need to stigmatize those who are made to instantiate the bad term of this relationship.

The idea of the will does not invite an understanding of subjective life, indeed the reverse. Conceived as will, individuality centres on the capacity of the adult individual to rule his or her internal life by means of the disciplines of the will. As others (Rose 1999; Heyes 2007) have demonstrated, the unruly and sometimes chaotic inner world of the individual is transformed into an orderly basis of conduct through submitting it to norms that the self imposes on itself. The normative regime of the will in fact invites the reduction of the complexity of subjective life that takes the form of splitting it into that which can be acknowledged and known as normatively-oriented conscious intention, and that which has to be placed under the rule of such conscious intention. The notion of the self-disciplined individual who voluntarily assumes externally prescribed normative obligations that provide the scaffolding of his or her self-rule is an older idea than that of the self, and it is worth pausing to reflect why it is that the trend in contemporary social policy has been to retrieve the older idea of the will rather than that of the self. It is the idea of the will that undergirds the adoption of workfare policies as well as the imposition of mandatory treatment regimes on people who are mentally ill, deemed to be lacking in an effective capacity for self-government, thus justifying others in imposing treatment norms on them. My sense is that the elaboration of the idea of the self as the subject of social policy, bringing with it as it has a sense of the complexities of subjective life, has also incited a desire to cut through and simplify such complexity. This desire is expressed in a re-articulation of the disciplines of the will, now associated not just with male householders but with all adults on a non-discriminatory basis. I return to the idea of the will in social policy in Chapter 5, and show how it undercuts a public ethic of subjective life by organizing welfare as the essentially private responsibility of the individual considered in terms of the idea of the will.

A right to self-preservation

When a mother calls her baby into psychological being as a self, she is inviting her baby to assume existence alongside her, his other parent, and still others beyond the parental couple, as a self in their live company. The mother is facilitating the psychological birth of the baby as a subject or self who can communicate with other selves. In so doing, the mother might be said to be preserving, as well as facilitating the actualization, of a potential for selfhood that is already there. Bollas (1989, 11) says of this potential: 'it is enough to say that infants, at birth, are in possession of a personality potential that is in part genetically sponsored and that this true self, over the course of a lifetime, seeks to express and elaborate this potential through formations in being and relating'. In a somewhat different formulation building on Winnicott's conception of the spontaneous gesture as the manifestation of the true self, Bollas (1989, 9) says:

> [For Winnicott] The true self was aliveness itself, and, although he saw it as an inherited potential, he did little to extend this understanding of the concept. If we are to provide a theory of the true self … it is important to stress how this core self is the unique presence of being, that each of us is; the idiom of our personality.

It may seem odd to harness seventeenth-century language of self-preservation to the notion that the elaboration of the potential of the individual to assume life as a self requires the facilitation of particular others and the facilitation of a public culture that is oriented to knowledge of the subjective vicissitudes of living life as a self. Yet it is in seventeenth-century civil philosophy that we find the discovery of a fundamental insight: it is the right to self-preservation that is found-ational of all other rights for if one is not alive as a self, one cannot enjoy any other right associated with freedom to be and act as a self. On this basis, we can understand relationships that are oriented to the welfare of the self as relationships that are oriented to its preservation. When such preservation involves work on behalf of the growth of the self, it is still the preservation of 'a personality potential' and its trans-mutation into manifest elaborations of the self that is at issue.

The idea of self-preservation directs our attention to what it is to be a self in a way that the idea of the will does not. With self-preservation, we have to attend to the question of what it means for the subject to experience itself as a self. The idea of the will empties the self of its substantive complexity and unconscious dynamics and requires the subject to be present only in its conscious intention, desire, or deliber-ation. It makes no sense to speak of the preservation of the will. All that the will demands is that its jurisdictional force and reach be recog-nized by other wills. Hegel (1991) termed the right to exist as will 'abstract right'. He had in mind the way in which the will *qua* will can be expressed as any and all forms of desire or choice while being limited by none of these. In a real sense, it is of no consequence that my will is expressed in this choice, while your will is expressed in that one; all that matters in this way of thinking about the subject is that each of us is free to choose. When we turn our attention to the subject thought of as a self, we have to consider the subject in her substantive uniqueness, shaped as this is by how she was parented, how she has articulated her personality potential, by her relationships with significant others, by her social-economic positioning, and by a cultural-historical horizon of life experience that she shares with some of her contemporaries.

Subjective right as the right to self-preservation

In her book *The State and the Rule of Law,* the French republican polit-ical theorist, Blandine Kriegel rightly argues that the idea of human rights is not new; it has a history that goes back, she proposes, to an early modern idea of the individual as entitled to what she calls sub-jective rights. Essentially, she argues that this is an idea of how rela-tionships between human beings should be conducted so that they respect and value 'the right of each person to his own body, the right to life' (Kriegel 1995, 35). Subjective rights concern the right of each individual to be alive as the individual that her or she is, and, thus, to be free to conduct her life so that it expresses her individuality. Subjective rights concern *status libertatis* which has to do with 'liberty and personal security, the right of each person to his own body, the right to life' (Kriegel 1995, 35). The right to self-preservation is foundational of all other rights. That is, all other rights have to refer back to subjective rights as their ground. If it should turn out that other rights, either in their conception or in their exercise, contradict subjective rights, these other rights have accordingly to be revised so that they are consonant with subjective rights. Thus, to use an obvious example, both the conception and the exercise of property right have to be consonant with subjective right. This would be true also of political and civil rights.

In a previous discussion of subjective right understood as the right of each human being to self-preservation (Yeatman 2007b), I propose that 'the idea of self-preservation turns on the valuing of each human being as a self':

> In order to be a self, the human being has to be alive in both the organic and the subjective senses of being alive. Thus valuing each human being as a self means valuing whatever conduces to the quality of being alive of the self as an embodied subject (Yeatman 2007b, 107).

I continue to say:

> Once examined, the idea of self-preservation can be seen to denote a set of relationships that bring together (a) what is involved in the subject being alive as a self, (b) what is involved in the subject being in the 'live company' (Alvarez 2002) of other selves, and (c) what it is that others, both as particular selves and as a political society of selves, have to do in order that the status claim to be a self is made possible. Freedom is intrinsic to the idea of self-preservation for the claim to be a self centres on the notion that one should be free to engage in life in one's own way so that one's life becomes one's own. The term self-preservation highlights what usually goes unremarked: the intrinsic coupling of freedom and life (Yeatman 2007b, 108).

The idea of self-preservation implies other ideas; together they constitute the complex of meaning that this idea involves. If we open up this complex of meaning we find five interlocking ideas. The first of them is the positive ethical conception of the individual human being as a self; this is the idea of subjective rights. The second idea is a negative one: the subject can enjoy life as a self only if she is not treated as a slave. Early modern political thinkers associated the master-slave relationship with the private discretionary right of the master of the household over his slaves. At core, slavery means the subjection of the individual to the arbitrary will of another. As other contemporary republican thinkers (Quentin Skinner 1998, Chapter 1; Philip Pettit (1997, 2002) clarify, the point is not that the slave may be lucky enough to have a master who is kind, benign, and generous; rather it concerns the status of the subject who is a slave. The status of the slave inherently exposes this individual to the arbitrary will of the master:

> While such slaves may as a matter of fact be able to act at will, they remain at all times in *potestate domini*, within the power of their masters. They accordingly remain subject or liable to death or violence at any time ... The essence of what it means to be a slave, and hence to lack personal liberty, is thus to be *in potestate*, within the power of someone else (Skinner 1998, 41).

Philip Pettit calls the condition of being 'within the power of someone else' domination. He argues that there are two respects in which domination is to be considered as antagonistic to freedom. Firstly, when someone is subject to another's domination, it creates 'a specific kind of uncertainty' in the former: 'The person who is subject to the arbitrary will of another will never be sure of where they stand or what to expect, and so may find it difficult to make firm plans; after all, any plans they make will be hostage to the will of the master' (Pettit 2002, 350). Secondly, a relationship of domination involves an inherent and 'characteristic asymmetry of status'. Pettit (2002, 350) argues that everyone will know that the person who is dominated cannot speak or act for herself without risking the dominator's ill favour or wrath. Accordingly, others outside this relationship cannot ascribe him or her a voice that claims their attention and respect; they cannot be sure when s/he speaks that it is what s/he really feels and thinks or is simply the voice of his or her compliant adaptation to the dominator's will.

   This is an issue of relevance in many welfare service settings, especially those where people are totally dependent on how others organize their everyday living environment, and, in addition, where these are people whose level of cognitive impairment makes it difficult for them to assert their own interests. In a nuanced discussion of how normal people, in a gesture of psychic defence against knowledge of loss, pain and trauma, pressure those who have suffered these things to smile, and 'keep happy', Valerie Sinason (1992, Chapter 6) discusses very ordinary dynamics of domination to which babies, children who are handicapped, and other vulnerable people are subject. She talks of 'the handicapped smile' as the compliant adaptation that these individuals are required to make to the wishes of their more powerful others:

> People who are close to great grief and cannot bear it encourage 'happiness' and smiling. Old people's homes and wards as well as homes for the mentally and multiply handicapped are victims of this. Lily Pincus ... described a beautifully kept hospital where the Matron said, 'And here you see our darling babies.' The old women were spotlessly dressed. 'They were all smiling because that is what is expected of "darling babies" but in contrast to babies they were not allowed to risk any attempt at independence (Sinason 1992, 141)'.

Sinason's psychoanalytically informed awareness shows how readily, and for very human emotional reasons, the more powerful subject can invite compliance rather than the unfolding of his or her personality potential in the dependent subject. Sinason is interested in how workers interact with people who are 'mentally handicapped': 'Being close to something that has gone wrong is a permanent reminder of the frailty of the human body and mind' (Sinason 1992, 208). If service workers are not supported in dealing with their own feelings, and in the time-taking work of providing meaningful personal contact to highly dependent people in institutions, group homes and other service settings, they will readily engage in a relationship of domination over these individuals:

> The reasons for this state of affairs vary. The depression of the powerless, speechless patient can pass into the medical or social work hierarchy barely touched. Poor pay and conditions can mean that the most deprived are tended by the almost equally deprived, who are then envious of the 'care' their clients get. 'No-one mops up after me,' protested one nursing assistant. These dummies have the time of their life just sitting down eating, pissing and shitting, knowing that I have to clean it all up.' In one unit I observed, staff rushed the 'residents' through their unchosen lunch to make sure of their own free time. The unit was small and was supposedly a first

step in the 'return to the community'. However, the kitchen was clearly for staff only and so was the right to change television channels and set the time for bed (Sinason 1992, 208–209).

Contrary to the Stoic idea that an individual who is positioned as a slave can retain an inner sense of self into which they can retreat in the face of external denial of their sense of self, Sinason shows how such external denial enters into the internal organization of the self. She suggests that sometimes the 'handicapped smile' is adopted by the individual concerned as not just an external defence but an inner one. She mentions 'an obese, severely multiply handicapped boy of 13 at the beginning of an assessment':

> Andy was blind, hemiplegic and epileptic. His school said that he was very happy, he smiled all the time, it was just that he masturbated in assembly. I visited him in a small classroom the school provided for such visits. I said my name was Mrs Sinason and his teachers had asked me to come because they felt he was feeling quite sad lately. That, I am afraid, was a lie! His teachers had said that he was happy. With a very guttural accent he said 'No. Happy. Happy all time.' There was a huge clown-like smile on his face as he said those words. 'Happy all the time?' I asked. 'Yes.' 'Happy when you have a fit?' There was a long pause. Then he opened his mouth, paused; the huge smile returned. 'No. But happy all the time.' I repeated that he was not happy when he had a fit but he was otherwise happy. 'Yes', he said happily on safe ground again. 'Happy about being in a wheelchair?' I asked. Then his face changed and became more serious. 'No,' he said emphatically. He sat up in the wheelchair. 'No. Not happy. Sad. Angry. I'm sad and I'm angry.' Speech, ability, language knowledge, grammatical structure, feeling, all improved immediately it was made clear that the false happy self was not required (Sinason 1992, 142).

Here we see Sinason creating a facilitating environment where it is both possible and safe for Andy to engage and own his subjective experience, without which he cannot enjoy a freedom for his sense of self, however painful the feelings that such freedom brings with it. Sinason comments elsewhere in her book:

> In working with the mentally handicapped, we know we are dealing with trauma. However, there is another unthinkable thought. It is

that they have emotional intelligence: somewhere they know and understand what is happening within and around them. Once that thought is bearable to the client, the client senses that growth is possible. In a similar way, if an institution provides privacy clients will know that they have the possibility of such space. The emotional space in a worker is matched by the architectural space of the building (Sinason 1992, 214).

The third idea that belongs to the complex of ideas involved in positing the individual as a subject of right is also a negative one: it is unethical to treat an individual as a thing. Kriegel (1995, Chapters 1, 2 and 3) discusses how early modern theorists of subjective rights argue against feudalism on this ground. In a feudal relationship, the lord has mastery over all that falls within his jurisdiction or *dominium*. This is his private domain to do with as he pleases; here we can see the close relationship between the feudal right of private *dominium* to the right of the master to control the slave. Each involves a private discretionary right over that which the lord or master is said to rightfully command as belonging to him. In this respect, each is a form of the assertion of property right.

The fourth idea is the proposition that subjective right is possible only as it is named, upheld, and secured as a matter of *public* right. It is not a private, discretionary matter, but a question of the ethical nature of how human beings regard and relate to each other. This is an inherently public issue. Thus Pufendorf (cit Kriegel 1995, 26) argues, moral beings 'are not things like physical beings; "they only possess each other by means of institutions"'. It is here that the precise objection to the subjection of human beings to the power of private property resides. As Kriegel (1995, 26) puts it, the fundamental objection against feudalism is that it 'confuses public relationships among individuals with the private relationships between a human being and a thing, treating persons as goods. Now Pufendorf's meaning becomes clear when he says that moral beings 'only possess each other by means of institutions'. If people are to relate together on the basis of reciprocal recognition of subjective right, this is a public relationship which has to be institutionalized as such. The institutional form of such a relationship is the sovereign state under law, a state that functions as a public authority (Locke's phrase), where offices cannot be bought and sold, but are designed and allocated in terms of public principles of accountability to a law that secures subjective right. One such principle is the 'impartial' or non-discriminatory treatment of those who come under the jurisdiction of the public authority.

The fifth idea concerns the nature of the state as the public authority. If the state is to function in this way, it cannot be a state that in its *modus operandi* is oriented to war, or *imperium*, for such a state by its nature threatens the right to self-preservation. Kriegel (1995, 21) argues, 'The early modern jurists sought to distinguish sharply between sovereign power and imperial power, so as to show that the sovereign state is not a creature of war but rather of peace, and it prefers the pacific negotiation of rights to the clamour of arms'. I might add that a state that allocates a considerable proportion of its revenue to the advancement of its military might is not one that is likely to make the kinds of allocation that are necessary to secure the self-preservation either of those who come under its direct jurisdiction or who fall within its sphere of imperial influence.

The opening of a relational space for the articulation of the self

Where the individual is conceived as will, the jurisdictional space for the exercise of her will is private in nature; it is boundaried so that it separates this individual's jurisdiction of the will from that of others. Of course, a boundary is a form of relationship, but in this case the function of the relationship is to separate individuals and to keep each of them attendant on their own respective business. When it is the individual as a self that is in view, it is important that the individual have space sufficient to permit her freedom to explore possibilities of personality elaboration, but in this case this space does not exclude others. Rather it concerns the conduct of relationships between subjects as selves able to recognize each other as both distinct and connected. They have to inter-relate in such a way as to create an opening for each of them to articulate their sense of self. Whether it is the mother who tunes her being into the baby's rhythms and expressions of being, thereby opening a relational space within which the baby can come to enjoy what Winnicott called a continuity of being, or adult partners and friends who actively invite and facilitate through listening the other's articulation of self experience on a reciprocal basis, the space for the expression of the self is internal to the relationship. Such space demands not separation but a form of active practice of co-existence.

In fact, this was how Émile Durkheim (in *The Division of Labor in Society*) conceived individualization. He spoke of individualization in terms of a space that opens up within social organization for the expression of individual differences. This is a fundamental insight that is too often lost in the assumption still made by many that individualism is antagonistic to the social. Rather it is a profound modulation of the social, of which there can be two such kinds: individualization *qua* will; individualisation *qua* self. Durkheim offered his own critique of individualisation *qua* will precisely because this is a way of thinking about the individual that brackets the social in relation to the assertion of the will; it is invested in assuming rather than explaining all the ways in which the assertion of the will depends on a prior education and co-temporal forms of public regulation.

The opening of a relational space for the expression and articulation of individual differences has to occur within all the modalities of social life: within language and cultural expression, the architectural design of space, occupational and civic life, as well as the conduct of relationships of service delivery, care, parenting, educating, and governing. Such regard for the human being as a self is articulated in what both people and their institutional order have to do in order to open up a relational space where it is safe for each human being to articulate his or her unique sense of being in the world, and where, in addition, such self articulation informs how both this individual's fellows and the institutional order interact with him or her. Consider how conversation, deliberation, decision making, teaching and learning have to be conducted if within these social practices there is to be space for the expression of individual difference. Instead of a hierarchical conception of an authoritative leader for these relational contexts who directs conduct, those who may have more knowledge (information, experience, and wisdom) than others have to offer it in a way that invites others to be present as individuals who have their own sense of being in the world. Those who have expertise also have to use it to actively facilitate an open conversational relationship between them and those to whom they offer their expertise where it is possible for the latter to question the nature and relevance of this expertise as it is offered in the particular context of this relationship in the here and now. Thus in its offering, knowledge has to be both contextualized and adapted to the individuality of those to whom it is offered.

More generally, the opening of a relational space for the expression of individual differences means that in any interaction, and as appropriate to differences in maturity, capability and authority, all people have to take responsibility for inviting their fellow participants to be present as individuals with their own unique ways of apprehending the world. As Iris Marion Young argued, in relation to her conception of communicative democracy, the first step always in inviting one's fellows to be co-present is the welcoming of their presence. She sees this as a political act, an act that she calls greeting. She explains:

> At that most basic level, 'greeting' refers to those moments in every-day communication where people acknowledge one another in their particularity. Thus it includes literal greetings, such as 'Hello', 'How are you?', and addresses people by name. In the category of greeting, I include also moments of leave-taking, 'Good-bye', 'See you later', as well as the forms of speech that often lubricate discussion with mild forms of flattery, hugs, the offering of food and drink, making small talk before getting down to business (Young 2000, 57–58).

Prior to turning to the content of what is to be transacted between subjects, there is a process of subject-to-subject or of what Bollas (1993, 23) would call idiom-to-idiom recognition: 'Prior to a thought to be conveyed, a world to refer to, act in, and share is the gesture of opening up to the other person where the speaker announces "Here I am" for the other, and "I see you" (Young 2000, 58).'

Public protection of this space

If there is to be space available within the conduct of social relationships for the expression of individual difference, then there has to be protection of this space. Such protection, ultimately, can come only from the public authority or the state. It is only the state that can secure the right to have rights (Arendt 1975, Chapter 9). It is the role of the state to secure the status of the individual human being as a person by providing protection against want, domination, exploitation and abuse of the individual by others. Domination, exploitation and abuse are different expressions of the same phenomenon, when one individual deprives others of space within which to assume an existence in their own unique way and requires of these others that they exist only to serve his (or her) will.

If the state should operate as the public authority that articulates and secures the ethical order of subjective rights, how does the state do this without articulating subjective rights as norms that individuals should impose on their own conduct? It is a contradiction in term for subjective rights to be converted into a normative doctrine that is then imposed on people. Donald Winnicott was concerned with this issue.

He thought it highly likely that many people in authority would use their power sentimentally in such a way as to convert freedom into a set of normative prescriptions for how people should act, think, and feel. Sentimentality occurs, Winnicott proposed, when people are unable to accept their own internal complexity, specifically their hatred and, more generally, what he calls their personal awfulness.[2] He argues that it is crucial that mothers and professionals charged with the care of others acknowledge their hatred of them: of their dependent neediness, their inability to grant the carer an independent existence and to appreciate her point of view, their ruthless self-concern, their seeming lack of gratitude, and so on. If hatred is acknowledged, then it does not have to be unconsciously acted out. More to the point here, if hatred is acknowledged, if indeed the enormous difficulty each one of us has in being a self who is capable of recognizing others as selves is something we can come to intimately know in our selves, then we will not convert the challenge of living ethically into moral prescriptions that we impose on others.[3] Instead we are likely to recognize in others our own difficulties, and to be clear that no one can grow through being forced to comply with externally imposed injunctions.

Winnicott emphasized the importance of the mother in the first instance, the parents in the second, being free to find what it is to be good-enough providers of a facilitating environment in which the baby can learn to be, and to organize its being as, a self. This comes out clearly in the example that Davis and Wallbridge use of his work to show what he means. They are citing a lecture on the subject of breast-feeding to members of the National Childbirth Trust, it being as clear then as it is now that breast-feeding, conditions permitting, is preferable to feeding by the bottle. Winnicott emphasizes the way in which breastfeeding engages both mother and baby in their respective capacity for 'sensuous coexistence' (Winnicott cit Davis and Wallbridge 1981, 155), where their being alive to and in each other's presence builds a rich and mutually nourishing relationship. Here is the segment of the lecture that clearly indicates Winnicott's desire to stay clear of sentimental moral prescription:

> What I want to do first is dissociate myself from a sentimental attitude towards breast-feeding. There is no doubt whatever that a vast number of individuals in this world today have been brought up without having had the experience of breast-feeding. This means that there are other ways by which an infant may experience physical intimacy with the mother ...

I have seen a great number of children who were given a very bad time with the mother struggling to make the breast work, which of course she is completely unable to do because it is outside her conscious control. The mother suffers and the baby suffers. Sometimes great relief is experienced when at last bottle feeding is established and at any rate something is going well in the sense that the baby is getting satisfied by taking in the right quantity of suitable food. Many of these struggles could be avoided if religion were taken out of this idea of breast-feeding. It seems to me the ultimate insult to a woman who would like to breast-feed her child, and who comes naturally to do so, if some authority, a doctor or a nurse, comes along and says 'You must breast-feed your baby'. If I were a woman this would be enough to put me off. I would say: 'Very well then I won't'.

Thus leaving aside the importance of the state imposing the law on those who break the law, the question of how the state uses its authority to cultivate a capacity for ethical life is an important one. Winnicott emphasizes the state's role in providing a boundary for a space within which people can exercise their freedom and grow through such practice. It is important that the state provide information and non-intrusive support to people especially in their parenting (and other carer) roles. In providing a boundary, the state also is a specific bounded community, thus permitting those who are within it to address the particularities of challenges for good-enough democratic co-existence on terms that make sense for this specific political community, given its history, geo-political positioning, and internal political ecology.[4] Winnicott is suggesting that a central role of the stable democratic state is to *trust* people to do whatever it is they are to do in good-enough ways so that, by the gift of this trust, people can learn to use their freedom constructively, to learn from their forays into 'creative living', and to contribute that learning to the larger societal set of public conversations. On this understanding of the state, it is clear that, under normal circumstances, public policy needs to be designed from the point of view of facilitating what 'ordinary, good' people (Winnicott's 1986, 247, phrase for 'ordinary, good parents') are already doing, not from the point of view of managing and controlling what he calls 'antisocial' people. Essentially, then, Winnicott is suggesting that the state should function so as to provide a facilitating environment for a nationally-bounded society.

On this approach, we can understand more readily why litigious 'rights' based approaches to implementing the status of the person in the case of individuals who are vulnerable to discrimination and stigma are not all that effective (see Young and Quibell 2000; Sayce 2003; Nedelsky 1993). To put it simply: people cannot be made to be ethical. Of course the law needs to be implemented. For example, anti-discrimination law is critical to ensure that people with disability have effective rights not to be discriminated against especially within the workplace. However, as Liz Sayce (2003) emphasizes, a point that is also central to John Braithwaite's work on regulation, it is more important to use the power of the state to facilitate compliance than to engage in litigation against law-breakers: 'The success of a law is determined not by the number of legal cases brought under it, but by the rate of compliance' (Sayce 2003, 631). Litigation should be combined with method of persuasion and conciliation as ways of enforcing the law (Sayce 2003, 633); Braithwaite (e.g. Braithwaite and Makkai 1994) argues that litigation should be the point of last resort, it being far more important to develop a culture of educated compliance with the law within say the industry of nursing home proprietors. Sayce discusses the important of educating public awareness about what constitutes discrimination and how it can negatively affect people. Again, it is important that such education proceed non-doctrinally and non-sentimentally.

Notes

1 Victoria Climbié died on 25 February 2000 when she was eight years old. She was 'systematically tortured and then murdered by her aunt and her aunt's partner in North London' (Cooper and Lousada 2005, 145). Between April 1999 and the time of her death she 'was known to a wide range of services including two housing services, four social services departments, and two police child protection teams (Cooper and Lousada 2005, 149)'. The Victoria Climbié Report was the outcome of an inquiry led by Lord Laming. Cooper and Lousada direct their attention to whether this report was able to adequately integrate the systems-focused procedural and process issues of child protection work, as they came up in relation to this case, with the emotional challenge of thinking about painful things: 'this work requires us to think about painful things. If we can manage it, then it is a kind of learning that can lead to growth (Cooper and Lousada 2005, 150)'. They suggest that the genre of the public inquiry report does not conduce to such learning (see Cooper and Lousada 2005, 151–152).

2 'Sentimentality, according to Winnicott, is a quality born of the repression of hate—of the inability to admit anywhere in himself or herself that he or she is capable of hating' (Davis and Wallbridge 1981, 123). Davis and Wallbridge refer to the long list of reasons Winnicott (1992, 201) gives in 'Hate in the Counter-transference' for why it is that the mother hates her baby.

3   'The truly responsible people of the world are those who accept the fact of
     their own hate, nastiness, cruelty, things which co-exist with their capacity
     to love and to construct' (Winnicott cit. Davis and Wallbridge 1981, 150).
4   Winnicott (1986, 256) makes two provocative remarks on this point: 'It is
     not possible for persons to get further in society-building than they can get
     with their own personal development'. And—'If the whole world were our
     society, then it would need to be at times in a depressed mood (as a person
     at times inevitably has to be), and it would have to be able fully to acknow-
     ledge essential conflict within itself. The concept of a global society brings
     with it the idea of the world's suicide, as well as the idea of the world's
     happiness. For this reason we expect the militant protagonists of the world
     state to be individuals who are also in a manic swing of manic-depressive
     psychosis'.

4
The Self as the Subject of Welfare

If we wish to be free to live our lives so that they are expressive of our sense of self, then our relationships with others have to function so that they support us in this freedom. The mode of living that is that of the self is always a complex set of dynamics involving the relationships of the self both to its external environment and its internal environment, where there is a complex and often faulty feedback loop between these two relationships. While a well-functioning self is open to adapting the ways in which it acts (thinks, feels, moves, and senses) in relation to changes in its external environment, if it is stuck in internal patterns of past adaptation to an environment that no longer presents, then it is not free to engage openly and creatively with his or her current environment.

Where the individual has already achieved a sense of self through the good fortune of experiencing good-enough parenting, and has the internal and external resources to go on to shape his or her life so that it enables him or her to explore his or her sense of self, for the most part, s/he can arrange her relationships to others so that they nourish, facilitate and support his or her sense of self. Where s/he cannot do this—for example relationships at work, in service transactions, and so on—s/he has the inner resources to contain the suffering these relationships cause him or her and to think about whether s/he needs to change these aspects of his or her life. The simple truth is that s/he is able to use the relational space that has opened up in the kind of society s/he lives in for getting on with living her life as the self that s/he is. Until, of course, catastrophe of one kind or another strikes: his or her marriage breaks down, s/he has an accident which causes him or her to be severely disabled, s/he develops a serious life-threatening illness, s/he loses his or her job and has to go onto public income support. Now s/he is in a position where other people have the power to profoundly affect his or her sense of self: both how s/he feels about him or herself as this is affected by how other people treat him or her, and the degree of freedom s/he feels in shaping his or her life to reflect his or her sense of self. This position describes all people who are dependent for their quality of life and life chances on welfare services.

In this chapter I explore three aspects of what it is to be a self in relation to what others have to do in order to facilitate the coming into being and sustaining of each of these. The first aspect concerns the organization of the subject as a self with its own distinctive integrity. I call this the integrity of the self and it is orientation to this aspect of the self that invites others to view the subject as a whole person. The second aspect concerns the ability of the self to independently act: I call this the independence of the self. When others facilitate or assist the independence of the self, they acknowledge the importance of independence to the status of the individual considered as a person. The third aspect concerns the ability of the subject as a self to accept, observe and reflect on her sense of self. I call this ability self-awareness, and I see this as the foundation of such self determination as it is possible to have. Self-awareness has to be facilitated by others, and when they do this they are positively assisting and facilitating that aspect of personhood that is implicated in the project of freedom understood as self-determination.

My argument is that when it is the self that is the subject of welfare, the service delivery relationship has to be conceived as a relationship of facilitation of each of these three aspects of selfhood. In this way the service delivery relationship enters into the constitution of the status of the individual as a subject of right—as a person.

The integrity of the self

The integrity of the self refers to what Winnicott called the unit status of the self. This refers to the achievement of a fundamental level of self-organization that permits the subject in question to integrate the thinking, feeling, sensing and moving aspects of its being into a single centre of subjective experience. When this occurs the subject is then able to identify as the 'I' that is the centre of these different aspects of experience. The subject is ready to engage in what Christopher Bollas (1993) calls self experience.

The achievement of unit status is a developmental process which has gone well or well enough. It depends on the provision of what

Winnicott called good-enough maternal care to the new-born baby which can be provided, of course, by someone other than the biological mother of the baby. The mother provides a facilitating environment where she uses her own maturity as a self to meet the baby's psychological and physiological needs in an integrated fashion. When she physically holds the baby she is also emotionally communicating her love and care for the baby as well as her cognitive appreciation of, and wonder at, this baby as a new person who has arrived in her world. As Winnicott (1990, 49) put it, 'Holding includes especially the physical holding of the infant, which is a form of loving'. The 'holding' the good enough mother provides is reliable and responsive to the unique being of this baby: 'it includes the whole routine of care throughout the day and night, and it is not the same with any two infants because it is part of the infant, and no two infants are alike' (Winnicott 1990, 49). Winnicott argued that it is within the environment of being held by its mother that the baby is able to 'build up what might be called a *continuity of being* (Winnicott 1990, 54)'. On this basis, the infant is now ready to integrate the different aspects of its existence so that they are experienced as emanations of its own I-ness. From here it is possible for the baby to learn to differentiate me and not-me which is expressed in a sense of here I am inside my skin, and others outside my skin are not me.[1] It is at this point that unit status is achieved.

The coming into existence as an integrated centre of subjective experience of the baby, then, is completely dependent on the availability of someone who offers good enough care to the baby. A sense of self depends, then, on the achievement of this fundamental level of subjective integration. If it is not achieved in infancy, owing to either constitutional or environmental failure, or both, it can be achieved, at least to a significant degree, later with intensive psycho-therapeutic provision of care. This is discussed at length by Alvarez (2002) who points out that the achievement of unit status in Winnicott's sense depends on the internalization of a good (psychic) object, one that enables the subject to feel at home with itself. Here she draws particularly but not only on the work of Wilfred Bion (see also Ogden 2008). Bion (1994) argued that a central function of the maternal environment, to use Winnicott's language, is to provide containment for the baby's unbearable feelings (rage, distress, anxiety). The mother is present to her baby in such a way that she psychically contains these feelings, and makes it possible for the baby to bear and think about them, remembering here that we are talking about unconscious processes of inner life. Only then can the baby 'have' these feelings and

allow them to enter into its experience; otherwise, without such containment, the baby has to fragment its experience, thus denying itself the
possibility of gathering experience into its sense of self, and, then, learning from its experience. If it cannot 'have' its experience, the baby cannot
come into being as a centre of self experience. It is this sense of being
one's own centre that Alvarez emphasizes in work with autistic and borderline children. Alvarez draws on Anna Freud's idea of 'structuralisation
of the personality', a metaphor suggesting that first the subject's ability to
contain or house their experience has to be built first before it can begin
to engage with its experience in such a way as to learn from it.[2]

Once the house has been built, the subject is ready to engage in what
Bollas (1993) calls self experience.[3] In self experience, the subject is engaging in creative processes of attempting to make external reality realize its
subjective imagination and desires. It uses the object world (both things
and other people) as media of evoking and thus articulating its idiom or
way of being a self. In such self articulations, objects—both those we
select and those that arrive by chance—transform the self: 'When we
select any series of objects—such as listening to a particular record, then
telephoning a particular person, then reading from a particular book—we
transform our inner experience by eliciting new psychic textures that
bring us into differing areas of potential being (Bollas 1993, 4)'. This is
why in an earlier book Bollas emphasizes that the idiom of the person—
that which is distinctly his or her way of being in the world—'is not ... a
hidden script tucked away in the library of the unconscious waiting for
revelation through the word'; 'It is more a set of unique person possibilities specific to this individual and subject in its articulation to the nature
of lived experience in the actual world' (Bollas 1989, 9).[4] The object has
its own integrity so that when the subject uses the object in order to articulate its sense of self, there is a sense in which the object also 'plays' the
subject (Bollas 1993, 31). It is in this subjective engagement with the
object world that the self creatively engages with limits. Just where these
limits are to be found, and how they are to be understood, has no independent reality outside the processes of creative subjective engagement
with the object world. It is a discovery of reality that is mediated by self-
exploration and self-knowledge. This is why Winnicott, and Bollas after
him, call the area that is neither inner reality, nor external reality, but an
intermediate zone where both meet in the medium of the articulations of
the self, 'a third area of human living':

> ... the area available for manoeuvre in terms of the third way of
> living (where there is cultural experience or creative playing) is

extremely variable as between individuals. This is because this third area is a *product of the experiences of the individual person* (baby, child, adolescent, adult) in the environment that obtains (Winnicott 1989b, 107, emphases in the original).

It is of considerable consequence then whether the object world (both other people and things) is rich or impoverished in relation to the opportunities for self experience.

Bollas (1989, 9) suggests each individual needs a personal space that expresses its sense of self when he says: 'We are singular complexities of human being—as different in the make-up of our characters as in our physiognomies; our person design finds its expression in the discrete living villages (composed of all those objects we select to cultivate our needs, wishes, and interests) that we create during our lifetime'. The individual needs not just an external space within which its sense of self can find expression but also a sense of internal space (where it can dream, imagine, be lost in its own inner world). Such space can be easily compromised by others who have the power to shut down such external space (deprive the individuals of opportunities to creatively engage with the object world) or to invade the individual's inner space. As Bollas proposes, it is inevitable that the parental aesthetic overlay that of the individual's, but it is of consequence whether this is simply an overlay or a displacement of the individual's own aesthetic.

Every aspect of the integrity of the self depends on the active and positive presence of others who have the power either to facilitate this integrity or to interfere with its development and ongoing processes of maturation. This is true for people who are not dependent on welfare services; and it is true for people who are. The difference is that the former, at least if they are adults, are likely to have more discretion in choosing the others with whom they closely interact.

The independence of the self

It is of crucial importance to the individual that s/he be able to independently act on behalf of his or her sense of self, specifically, that s/he be able to act in order to realize his or her intention. Independence has two components: the intention to act on my own behalf, and the ability to carry out my intention. Thus, if I am to be independent in getting something down from a shelf, I need to be able to intend to reach for this object, and to be able to organize my movement so that I can reach for it. The quality of independence marks the individual's mode of engaging with her environment if it is both intentional and efficacious. Here we are talking again about self-experience through how the self engages with its environment but with the accent now on independence.

The capacity for independent action for some people can be exercised only with the assistance of others. Often such assistance takes the form of welfare services. The difference between people who can act independently without the assistance of others and those who can do so only with such assistance is real. The former have a freedom that is uncompromised by waiting on others to offer such assistance.

Where the individual can independently act (move, think, feel, and sense), it is important that the presence of others is not such as to interfere with the individual's independence. They have to give the individual space to exercise her independence, and to do this, they have to see the individual as separate from themselves. Where an individual is dependent on the assistance of others to carry out her intentions, she still needs others to give her space both in the forming and the expression of her intention as this carries over into a collaborative form of action, where it is the role of the others to lend their powers in such a way as to supplement her own. Her independence *is* compromised; but she can be assisted by others who lend their selves to enable her to be as independent as it is possible for her to be. This is how Winnicott positions the mother in relation to the baby; it is the mother who lends her powers to the baby to enable him to experience a sense of omnipotence, a sense of, the world is my oyster.

Where people are dependent on services either to supplement their powers and/or to build their capabilities for independent action, the critical importance of these services is obvious when it is clear that a sense of self demands expression in an independence of action. Where such independence of action is inherently compromised, it is important that the self in question be supported in coming to terms with such profound loss. Valerie Sinason (1992) discusses her work as a psychoanalytic therapist with a man experiencing progressive mental deterioration because of Alzheimer's disease. His was the progressive loss of intentionality, for the ability to form an intention depends on a capacity to think. Sinason (1992, 110) comments of the time a year before this man's death:

> He had held onto thinking as represented by my presence, as long as he could. According to his sons, therapy allowed him to come

to terms with his degeneration, with the unpicking of the fine embroidery that had been his brain.

Independence of action is a fundamental human freedom. This is something that Moshe Feldenkrais realized and built into his method of somatic education. It matters enormously whether I can get up from sitting to stand and then walk in a way that feels comfortable *and* within my own powers. Only then can I think that I would like to wander outside and enjoy the sensation of the sun on my skin. Strangely enough, some theorists who emphasize that individual autonomy needs the presence of others, and who talk about the relational aspect of autonomy, fudge the centrality of a capacity for independent action to autonomy. Thus Jennifer Nedelsky (1990, 180) advocates a conception of autonomy that does not require 'a separative self'; and Jeff Malpas (2007, 2) seems to suggest in the following statement that 'separation from others' is mutually exclusive of relationship to others: 'If the principles that determine human being are indeed principles of relationality that place human thinking and acting in an ever-present relation of interdependence with others and with the world, then to think and act autonomously will not be to think and act in separation from others and the world, but to think and act in a way that is attentive to them.'

It bears repeating then that independence of action is vital if individuals are to enjoy a sense of self, and that independence of action requires the positive presence of others in getting out of the individual's way, in separating themselves from this individual and letting her do her thing, and, as necessary, in positively lending their skills and powers to facilitating, building and supplementing the individual's own powers of independent action. Welfare service types that are oriented to facilitating an independence of action in individuals whose powers of independent action are compromised are of critical importance.

Self-awareness

Self-awareness refers to the ability of the self to observe itself, and, on the basis of such observation, to think, and, in the course of such thinking, to reflect on what it finds most meaningful as well as to ask whether it wants to continue to organize itself in the way that it does. Self-awareness is the basis of such self-determination as we can exercise. I cannot make or remake myself at will, but I can learn how to live with my limits, both those that are real, and those that turn out to be artefacts of my past experience, which I can change if I figure out how to do this. I have an inner world that is mostly unconscious, and which often erupts into action of mine that is mean, nasty, angry, enraged, envious, greedy and needy in relation to others. I can learn to come to terms with all aspects of my being, those that I like, those that I don't like, those that are constructive and those that are destructive, if I am able to endure the pain of knowing the difficult aspects of myself, in the process of which I can come to see that I am human after all, not the monster I feared myself to be.

Through self awareness we open up new possibilities of being a self in a world shared with other selves and other creatures. To practice self awareness means as I have said already a capacity to endure loss, to experience pain, and to accept limitation. It is in the experience of such loss, pain, and sense of limitation that new possibilities of being unfold because I am no longer paralysed by fear. I am able to step into a space of not knowing where I can begin to learn about possibilities of being both for myself and others.

The practice of self awareness has to be facilitated by others who already know something of this practice. Perhaps the core value of self awareness is that it permits us to think, rather than simply react, especially under conditions that we experience as a threat to our sense of self. The practice of self-awareness is one that opens up a quiet space within which the individual can listen to herself—thus the practice 'holds' a space within which self awareness can occur. The practice also in the sense intended by Bion provides a container for self experience so that the individual is able to bear difficult sensations, feelings, and thoughts, and then to think about them. We can think of the Buddhist practice of 'sitting', of Feldenkrais group and individual lessons, and of psychoanalytic use of 'free association' (see Bollas 2007), as different kinds of facilitated practice of self awareness.

There are many forms of practicing self awareness, some more rigorous than others. Every time someone asks us, 'what do you think', and is genuinely ready to wait for when and if we are ready to respond, as well as to listen carefully to our response, we are being invited to practice self awareness. In the work of Hannah Arendt, she borrows the figure of Socrates to emphasize the importance of someone playing midwife to our opinion (see also Fiumara 1990, especially Chapter 10). The Delphic injunction 'know thyself' means, Arendt (2005, 19) proposes, that I can 'understand truth' only by finding and engaging how the world is distinctively disclosed to me, and then by finding out how my 'opinion' is received by and relates to those of others. In practicing the art of maieutic or midwifery, Socrates 'wanted to help others give birth to what they themselves thought anyhow, to find the truth in their doxa':

> This method had its significance in a twofold conviction: every man has his own doxa, his own opening to the world, and Socrates therefore must always begin with questions; he cannot know before hand what kind of *dokei moi*, of it-appears-to-me, the other possesses. He must make sure of the other's position in the common world. Yet, just as nobody can know beforehand the other's *doxa*, so nobody can know by himself and without further effort the inherent truth of his own opinion. Socrates wanted to bring out this truth which everyone potentially possesses. ... The method of doing this is *dialegesthai*, talking something through, but this dialectic brings forth truth not by destroying *doxa* or opinion, but on the contrary by revealing *doxa* in its own truthfulness (Arendt 2005, 15).

Arendt suggests that an ability to open up an internal conversation of thinking, what she calls 'the two-in-one' practice whereby the self is able to consider it-self, is linked to the worldly experience of the plurality of opinions. Christopher Bollas advocates the psychoanalytic relationship as one where the analyst facilitates through listening the free association of the patient thus providing a space where the patient is able to listen to herself, and thus to experience this two-in-one dialogue (Bollas 1999, 21 where he makes explicit reference to this idea of Arendt).

The self as the subject of welfare

When the subject of welfare is understood to be the self, then welfare services have to be conceived, designed and implemented so that they support all three aspects of selfhood discussed in this chapter: the integrity of the self, the self's capacity for independent action, and the self's capacity for self-awareness. It is in this sense that welfare services and their mode of delivery are individualized. It is a different sense from that which occurs when the individual is thought of as will rather than as a self. I now turn to the conception of welfare services that follow on from the idea of the will as the subject of welfare.

Notes

1   'In favourable circumstances, the skin becomes the boundary between the me and the not-me. In other words, the psyche has come to live in the soma and an individual psycho-somatic life has been initiated' (Winnicott 1990, 61).

2   'First, as Anna Freud says, build the house; first, as Klein says, introject the good breast; first, as Bion says, you have to have an adequate container; first, as Bowlby says, have a secure base (Alvarez 2002, 117)'.

3   This is a rich development of Winnicott's conception of playing (see Winnicott 1989).

4   In his later book (Bollas 1993, 29–30) makes the same point slightly differently: '... I do not think of the self as phenomenologically unified. It cannot be, because in the first place, the true self is not an integrated phenomenon but only dynamic sets of idiomatic dispositions that come into being through problematic encounters with the object world. But these experiencings and the I's relation to them obviously yield senses of familiarity which allow us an illusion that the self is a unity. This sense derives ... from the continuous, reliable, and unconscious rapport between the I and the self's experiencings ...'

5
The Will as the Subject of Welfare—The Consumer Model of Service Delivery

Whether it is the North American idea of 'consumer-directed care' (Keigher 1999; Kapp 1997; Feinberg and Ellano 2000) or the British idea of 'user involvement' (Cowden and Singh 2007; Carr 2007; Scourfield 2005), there has been a remarkable shift in policy for the delivery of welfare services over the last decade. Instead of a professionalized relationship of service delivery embedded within the structure of public administration of publicly-funded welfare services, the model that prevailed up until the last quarter of the twentieth century, now the model is rhetorically shaped by the idea of consumer or service user 'choice', and, ideally anyway, such choice is to be assured through the natural development of a welfare service market.

Where consumers or service users are not wealthy enough to buy their own way into a service market, and remain dependent on public funds, there are two ways in which their access to services is subject to market principles. In the first of these ways, the consumer/user is given cash in hand by a public funding authority, and is empowered to buy the service she wants and needs. Depending on which particular scheme of 'consumer-directed care' (North America) or 'direct payments' (UK) we have in mind, it can be possible for someone else who lives with the consumer/user to be empowered as the purchaser of the home care package that is needed. As Keigher puts it in her (1999, 183) survey of 'consumer directed care' across a number of countries (Austria, Germany, Canada, and the United States): 'The policy strategy of consumer-direction or self-managed care is the granting of resources directly (or more directly) to the disabled person, or their surrogate, who makes his or her own decisions and choices, within the household or outside of it, about the services to obtain and to whom'. In the second way in which access to publicly-funded services is marketized, the government funding agency creates a 'quasi market' within which providers are asked to competitively tender for government-funded services for people who need welfare services. Funding is tied to 'outcomes' for particular individual service users, and there is usually some provision for giving service consumers/users 'choice' or at least right of exit in relation to providers. Here the government funding agency represents itself as the advocate of consumer/user choice by using a method of governance of service providers where funding is tied to the achievement of outcomes for individuals. The government makes proxy decisions on behalf of these individuals, and, so far as this is the case, the government assumes the role of consumer or customer.

Both ways of marketizing publicly-funded welfare services are guided by the economic ideal of the sovereign consumer who is free to choose the service she needs in a service market. Unlike a supermarket, however, where the consumer picks a product off the shelf, pays, and walks away, a welfare service involves an inter-subjective relationship that can last over considerable time depending on the nature of the need that is the basis of service provision. It is by means of the relationship that the service is delivered. In good part the quality of provision for client/user need will depend on the quality of the relationship as it will also depend on how well the service in question is resourced.

There are a number of major issues with this shift to a market-consumption model of service delivery and I shall briefly canvass several before I turn to the major issue that is the subject of this chapter: the discounting of the service delivery relationship that occurs when the service client is redesigned as a service consumer who asserts her preference or will in the service encounter. Before I indicate the bundle of issues that are inherent in this new approach to service delivery, I offer some historical context for why it has been adopted.

The historical context of the adoption of a market-consumption model of service delivery

In the 1970s and 1980s there was a convergence of three factors that moved the idea of service delivery in the direction of community care. The first of these factors was the decisive withdrawal of legitimacy from the older mode of institutional care for people with disabilities, mental illness, and frail older people. The second factor was the convenient and short-term view taken by relevant government agencies that community care would be cheaper than institutional care. They saw it as an opportunity to move away from the 'professional capture' of institutional care, to rely more on informal (family-based) systems of care, and, perhaps without thinking much about it, a way of offloading an expensive responsibility that had become highly politicized. It is fair to say that institutional closure proved to be the relatively easy part, the development of adequately resourced community services that are responsive to those who need them, the difficult part (see Bigby and Fyffe 2006 who distinguish between 'institutional closure' and 'deinstitutionalization').[1] After all, whatever the opportunistic motives of government departments and central financial agencies had been, this was a dramatic shift from an historically entrenched mode of care provision to an entirely new one that would take time to bed down, require policy and service innovation and new learning. The third factor, which contributed considerably to the delegitimation of the older method of institutional care, was the pressure from especially disability user movements 'for policies to support "independent living" and "empowerment" (Fernández *et al.* 2007, 98)'. It was from this direction that the idea of 'direct payments' (or, more broadly, individualized funding understood as giving the service user public funds to buy the service assistance she needs) came (see for the UK a much cited article by Jenny Morris 1997; and for the USA, Kendrick 2000). Advocates of individualized funding have tended to emphasize the importance of empowering the individual consumer/user, and a transfer of power away from bureaucratic and professional/provider dominance of the care system to the level of the individual consumer/user and her life world. Thus emphasis has been not so much on the reconfiguration of the triangular relationship between policy, provider, and client, as on a simple transfer of power, and a reduction of the triangular relationship to a dyadic one. Put another way, the model of power has been one of a zero-sum relationship (if they have it, we do not), not one of power sharing.

The radical idea of devolution of management of the care system to the level of the individual, sometimes with community-based infrastructural support for individuals as the employers of personal care workers, is part of the more general contemporary and 'anti-statist' (see Kriegel 1995) romance of 'civil society'. Local, community-based 'solutions' are understood to be better than state-sponsored and state-planned ones; government bureaucracy reductively conceived as so much 'red tape' and viewed as antagonistic to community-based initiative; and private sector firms are understood as more responsive to market demand than are professionalized services that have been embedded in a bureaucratized and 'statist' mode of service provision. Here we can see how highly-principled advocacy of individualized funding could come together with the opportunism of government departments in offloading historically acquired responsibilities in this context of anti-statist embrace of local community 'solutions'.

In the development of individualized funding approaches to community care, governments co-opted disability movement rhetoric. Scourfield (2007, 113–114) comments of Britain that: 'The disability movement's rights discourse, built around notions of empowerment, self-determination and societal change, has been successfully conflated with the New Labour vision to build an enterprise society.' He (2007, 114) comments further, 'This has allowed New Labor to re-deploy the technique of talking both to and for the people directly, in order to reprimand an "unresponsive" public sector'. Elsewhere, Scourfield (2005, 473) shrewdly comments, 'government has effectively sat its "market-consumer" discourse on the disabled movement's "social rights discourse", producing a powerful hybridisation but one riddled with tensions'.

The shift to individualized funding and community-based care approaches is symptomatic of a populist *zeitgeist*. Frank Riessman (1984, 2–3) with reference to the American context speaks of a new market consumerism that has become pervasive, a mentality 'that includes a demand for the new—for change, an appraising orientation, and some implicit power of choice'. He continues:

> Competing ads and claims get the consumer used to making choices—although not necessarily the best choices. But in a sense, consumers have been trained to scrutinize, question, compare, evaluate, check, appraise, shop and test. They come to experience the power that derives from choosing (Riessman 1984, 2–3).

Riessman (1984, 3) suggest that the ethos of market consumerism has proved to be contagious 'spreading its demanding, evaluative focus to issues and concerns other than market products'. He (1984, 3) concludes: 'This new consumer-based politics has a neopopulist bias—anti-big, anti-Washington, anti-bureaucratic, anti-elite, anti-expert, and anti-professional'.

Issues concerning a consumer-based model of delivering welfare services

There are a number of issues that are inherent in this model. I will briefly canvass two of them before I take up what I regard for our purposes as the central issue: the positioning of the service client as a service user or service consumer. The first issue concerns the ideological character of this populist model of service delivery. The second issue concerns the displacement of a public ethos and system of management of service delivery by a private one.

Populism has the singular virtue of appearing to cut through, and thus to reduce, the complexity of modern social arrangements by placing things within the direct control of the individual voter/consumer. Because it is an ideology wed to simplicity, rather than complexity, it deals in binaries: either professional dominance or consumer empowerment; either bureaucratized systems of service delivery or consumer-responsive ones; either equal partnership or paternalism, meaning an asymmetrical and hierarchical power relationship; either voluntarism or coercion (this binary for obvious reasons features strongly in mental health populist rhetoric); and, finally regarding the position of the client/user/consumer, either passivity or agency, a binary that semiotically engages the other central binary regarding the position of the person in relation to welfare services, either independence or dependence.

Thinking that is structured in terms of binaries—'either/or', not 'and'—is always ideological in the sense that it functions on behalf of commanding collective assent to values that are made to appear self-evident. It is fundamentally antagonistic to what Hannah Arendt called *selbstdenken*, both the capacity and the willingness to think for oneself, an inner conversation where the individual does not rely on 'preconceived categories' and moral rules, but engages in the unending activity of what she called understanding:

> Understanding, as distinguished from having correct information and scientific knowledge, is a complicated process which never produces unequivocal results. It is an unending activity by which, in constant change and variation, we come to terms with and reconcile ourselves to reality, that is, try to be at home in the world (Arendt 1994, 307–308).

When governments use ideological modes of thinking, they reduce complex concepts to buzz words that structure a sound-bite mode of communication with the public. For instance, 'user involvement' (in welfare policy and service delivery) is a complex concept that has been addressed as such in nuanced discussion by many analysts over the last 20 or so years (e.g. Beresford 2001; Pilgrim and Waldron 1998; Clark

1998) but it has been converted into an ideological mantra by the British New Labour Government. Cowden and Singh (2007, 6) remark:

'User involvement' is one of the central concepts in the strategy of 'reform' and 'modernization' of Public Services currently being led by New Labour. Whether one is talking about 'parent power' in education, the new 'patient-led' National Health Service, or the requirement that Social Care services place 'service users' at the centre of service provision, every government department is determined to remind those working across the public sector that the bad old days of statist paternalism are out—it is now the 'user who knows best'.

They comment further that it is inevitable that such a simplistic ideological deployment of a concept leads to lack of clarity and agreement as to what user involvement actually means. They suggest this idea 'really comes apart' when it implicates difficult service settings where people are subject to lawful coercion as in the case of mental health services, and we might add, other settings where professionals feel compelled to use their judgement to intervene in order to protect a vulnerable client from harm (see Clark 1998), not to say the much more delicate exchange I have discussed in Chapter 4 where it is the service professional's intervention that is the key to eliciting and facilitating the actual expression of what it is that the client wants.[2] Beresford (2001, 503) sees the deflection of the complex idea of 'user involvement' into populism as reflected in a more generalized emptying out of the substantive content and complexity of social policy: 'This is reflected in the significance attached to opinion and "message" polls, reliance on focus groups and emphasis on the presentation and language of policy rather than its detailed content and principles'.

This brings me to the second issue, or cluster of issues, I see as inherent in the adoption of a consumer-based model of welfare services. With this model the role of government is one of devolving decisions concerning the delivery of welfare services to the individual consumer in his or her life world. This is the 'enabling state', one that 'acts to facilitate private citizens "running their own affairs" rather than to embody public responsibility' (Cowden and Singh 2007, 12–13). As I have suggested already, such a simple model refuses to work with the inherently triangular and complex relationship between government as both policy maker and funding agency, service providers, and service clients (itself a complex category for it must include both the organized advocates of service clients, and the individuals themselves in the service transaction). Instead, government has the role of creating both ideological direction and institutional incentives for the creation of a series of service markets where the relationship is the simple one of service consumer exercising his or her preference in relation to the service market (choice of service and choice of provider).

As many commentators have observed, this model privatizes risk: risk management is devolved to the level of service delivery, to both providers and service clients/consumers (for an excellent discussion of this see I. Ferguson 2007). Social policy is reduced to the public management of an essentially private transaction, and, in this regard, social policy is no different from any other regulative policy with regard to the functioning of a private market. Such an approach to governing social policy not only privatizes the role of the welfare service client but it also privatizes the role of the welfare service provider. The public mission of the welfare service professions and service industries in developing services that secured the self-preservation of those who need them (see Chapter 2) is essentially cast aside, as is the responsibility of professional education and training institutions for the cultivation of a public professional service ethic and the responsibility of single providers for the training and supervision of workers. Within this framework it is not possible to create a public sphere of social policy within a particular area of need (disability for example) where the triangular relationship between service client advocates, service providers, and the government department can be openly practiced as a collaborative stakeholder approach to the development of policy, including the critical discussion of how funds can match needs. Public policy discussion is displaced by in-house government decisions about the allocation of funds and methods of controlling the performance of those now engaged at the front-line: in a quasi-market these are the service providers; in a direct payments context, these are the consumers. As Scourfield (2005, 480) points out that, with regard to direct payments, the role of government is a mixture of control and command, on the one hand, and *laissez-faire* on the other:

> ... with schemes such as direct payments, we see a policy where the managerialization of the self becomes both extended and 'deepened' by the requirement that the service user takes on more of the functions, risks and responsibilities which formerly would have been the remit of the state. This process ... requires that the service user not only manages themselves but that they also become the

manager of public funds, they agree to present their records for inspection and audit and, with the inputs they have been allocated, they assume responsibility for achieving agreed outcomes. Moreover, direct payments require more than the managerialization of the service user. It is assumed that service users will become more than managers—they should also be calculative risk takers and innovators. This means that their care or personal support will be 'what they make of it', no longer being arranged for them from public provision (Scourfield 2007, 116; and see also Scourfield 2005, 480).

I need add only that all commentators agree that the public resources sufficient to make care in the community effective for the different categories of welfare clients who need it have never been allocated. The tendency has been for resource scarcity to deepen, funding caps to be introduced, and for eligibility criteria to tighten (I. Ferguson 2007, 398; Bigby and Ozanne 2001 for a general cross-juridictional overview with regard to the service field of intellectual disability; Fernández *et al.* 2007, 116–117 present data for the British community care system that 'reveal a strong negative relationship between the per capita number of recipients of direct payments and the size of the average direct payment package'). Where the principle of rationing that is adopted is one of targeting the greatest need (Scourfield 2006, 9), there is a tendency for service allocation to be 'driven more by a response to crisis than an ability to provide preventative services before needs reach a high or urgent level (Bigby and Ozanne 2001, 185)'. In this context, as Keigher (1999) reminds us, those who are positioned as clients of publicly funded services, even when their position is reshaped to become that of a 'consumer', are very differently placed in relation to service markets than are those who are positioned as private clients with sufficient wealth of their own to purchase the services they consider they need. Notwithstanding the adoption of a rhetoric of consumer empowerment/user involvement, the former category are dependent on a level and quality of service that follows on the funds that government is prepared to allocate, while the latter category are not. As with schooling and health services, the adoption of a consumer model of welfare service provision leads to a class-based distinction between the quality and level of welfare services available to those who are dependent on direct public subsidy and those who can afford to buy into private care markets, but who are likely to get public subsidy in the form of fiscal welfare (tax relief).

The positioning of the welfare service subject as will

As is noted by many in these discussions, language is telling. The lingual repositioning of the welfare service client as customer, consumer or user indicates a profound reshaping of the relationship between the individual who needs a welfare service and the service provider. The welfare subject is to be present as 'will'. The service transaction and relationship are positioned as something that the welfare subject 'uses' or 'consumes'.

Rhetorically at least, the service transaction and relationship are to be directed by the welfare worker's choice or will. Where, as in the case of consumer directed care or direct payments, the individual welfare subject is also positioned as the employer of the care worker, the worker is subject to the employer's will as is the case with all employment relationships that come within the sphere of what is regarded as private property (the right of the employer to command what comes under the jurisdiction of his private will). A major unresolved set of issues in this type of care market is the question of the regulation of this relationship, the provision of training, and the protection of worker health and safety, adequate levels of pay and so on (this is discussed by Scourfield 2005 and 2007; Keigher 1999; Ungerson 1997). Regulation with regard to private employment relationships is always imposed from the outside by government as the public authority. Without regulation, private employment relationships are essentially left to the direction of the employer's will and, where relevant, to the employer's self-interest in retaining good employees.

In the service market model, the service deliverer—both the direct service worker and, where relevant, the service agent—are positioned as a means to fulfil the end, this being the will of the welfare service consumer. The service delivery relationship is instrumentalized on behalf of the will of the consumer. As with all expressions of consumer choice or preference—the assertion of will—the assumption is that the intentionality of the welfare subject can be encompassed in this way, as the conscious expression of what it is that one wills. Where people are unable to consciously express what it is that they want, the status entitlement of 'choice' falls away for this model does not permit an emphasis on how the service delivery relationship can facilitate the articulation of the service client's 'voice' and 'choice'. The consequence is that individuals, who for reasons of cognitive impairment, cannot manage a self-responsible conscious formulation of their wants/needs, drop out of the model; they have to be willed for by others, relatives, a case manager or some other professional. Thus the model of consumer-based welfare services authorizes a binary distinction between welfare subjects who can exemplify the power of the will, and those who cannot.

Let me say something more of this idea of will. 'Choice' is a labile concept; it can be used in different ways that implicate very different conceptions of how to structure relationships between a subject who chooses and other subjects. I have highlighted two ways: (a) the choice of the subject understood as the freedom of the will to express itself and to be carried out in appropriate action; (b) the choice of the subject understood as the freedom of the subject to express her sense of self such that it is articulated, listened to, and appropriately regarded within the relationships in which this subject finds herself. With choice understood as freedom of the will, in making his will the basis of his relationship to things and other subjects, as Hegel (1991, 75) puts it, these relationships acquire the subject's will as their 'substantial end'. Where relationships driven by the freedom of the will involve other people, there is a problem in reconciling the freedom of the will of one with the freedom of the will of another. There are only two modalities of relationship available: one that concerns an external relationship between wills typically expressed in 'contract' where each will agrees to recognize the other's private jurisdiction of willing as in this is my property, that is yours; the other is the internal relationship of the will to that which comes within its private jurisdiction, a relationship that is expressed as the unilateral freedom of the will's mastery or command over both things and other subjects. With choice understood as the freedom of the subject to express her sense of self, and to have her sense of self appropriately regarded in her relationships, these relationships are open to the expression of the sense of self of all those who participate in them. These relationships are multilateral and inter-subjective in nature. Where relationships directed by the will are simply hierarchical (the will commands), relationships between selves are not hierarchical but they can be asymmetrical as I discuss in the next chapter. Asymmetries of maturity, experience, skill and expertise may be central to the *raison d'être* of such relationships. However, such asymmetries do not in any way compromise the claims of the self in these relationships; rather they shape how these claims function as claims on an inter-subjective relationship. A good-enough parent does not negate the fact that her baby is immature and dependent on her care, but offers her care in such a way as to facilitate and support the developing sense of self of the baby. A professional does

not negate the fact that the service client is dependent on her expertise, but offers her expertise in such a way as to facilitate and support
the sense of self of the individual client.

The inadequacy of the consumer approach to the delivery of welfare services

The model of consumer will or choice assumes that the consumer
already possesses all the resources of rational decision making s/he may
need when it is more often the case that there is an inevitable asymmetry of competence and expertise in the relationship of the person who
needs a service and the service deliverer. Not just inevitable, but desirable; even in the case of a personal care service, it is desirable surely
that the personal carer have a minimum of competence, training in
standards of intimate personal care as well as those of occupational
health and safety, and knowledge of interactional boundary issues. The
consumer model of welfare service delivery is predicated on the denial
of such asymmetry, while the real question remains: how does this
asymmetry function, does it operate for or against the service user?

In their discussion of contemporary HIV-AIDS drug treatment regimes,
Race *et al.* (2001, 12) use the phrase 'consumerist understandings of the
clinic'. They are referring to the contemporary model of general practice medicine where the doctor sees her/his role as one of informing
the patient as to his/her options and then leaving it to the patient
to choose. The doctor thereby avoids what is viewed as paternalism;
s/he is not prescriptive but respectful of patient competence in choice
and decision making. The problem with this approach is that it does
not adequately respect the patient's subjective experience for it is the
nature of being a patient who needs medical expertise (especially when
serious and maybe life-threatening illness is at stake) to also need the
doctor to care about them as a person where such caring is informed
by the doctor's insight into their subjective experience, and, in turn,
informs how the doctor offers information to this individual so that
s/he can hear it, listen to it, and think about it. Information is thus
offered in a way that also facilitates the patient's subjective ability to
process and think about it (see Chapter 11). It is in how the doctor
does this that s/he provides containment for the patient's distress and
confusion in accepting that s/he is ill and may need treatment that
may be highly interventionist.

In an older type of general practice medicine, less reliant on scientific
testing for diagnostic purpose, and also less reliant on specialist referral,

the individual doctor is engaged in a complex process of integrating art and science in his professional judgement. Such judgement is always relative to the specificity of the context that is created by it being this particular individual in this particular social context who has this particular illness at a time when this range of treatment is indicated. While I am using the example of general practice medicine here, these remarks can be extended also to nursing, social work, occupational therapy, and psychotherapy, and also to what it is that a good personal carer provides in a community-based service setting. Martha Nussbaum offers an Aristotelian conception of the nature of such practical judgement. It is not so much the application of principles to a particular instance as it is the ability to allow the particular instance to guide one's perception and to invoke as the basis of judgement a highly complex and largely unconscious synthesis of prior knowledge, experience with other patients, and new learning in relation to this one. Nussbaum puts it in this way: it is a question of 'a confrontation with the situation itself, by a faculty that is suited to confront it as a complex whole'. She continues:

> General rules are being criticised here both for lack of concreteness and for lack of flexibility. ... Aristotle tells us that a person who attempts to make every decision by appeal to some antecedent general principle held firm and inflexible for the occasion is like an architect who tries to use a straight ruler on the intricate curves of a fluted column. Instead, the good architect will, like the builders of Lesbos, measure with a flexible strip of metal that 'bends to fit the shape of the stone and is not fixed' ... Good deliberation, like this ruler, accommodates itself to what it finds, responsively and with respect for complexity. It does not assume that the form of the rule governs the appearances; it allows the appearances to govern themselves and to be normative for correctness of rule (Nussbaum 1986, 301).

As far as the example of medicine goes, there is now something of a gulf that divides the medical specialist who applies scientific technique in surgery especially, and the general practitioner. Consider this statement from an HIV-treatments GP interviewed by Race *et al.* (2001, 13). The doctor is a high HIV-patient-caseload and gay GP working in inner Sydney:

> ... HIV GPs are sort of in that area between science and um—hopefully know patients very well and that's the nice thing with general practice ... you have to try and marry up scientific knowledge to the

psycho-social situation of the person ... I often see things where a patient I know very well has ended up at [name of a hospital] and one of the specialists has decided they are going to do blah, blah, blah with them and they come back here and I know that it's not going to work out because I know the person very well. And the specialist's only met them once for ten minutes ... I think it's very interesting because technically they know more than we do, but they don't know the patient nearly as well as we do.

... in general practice we may make the technical errors because we don't know the science as well, but I think the outcome may be better because we know the person. Which is a luxury, I suppose, of knowing a person very well.

The problem with the consumer model of service delivery is that it shifts responsibility for decision making to the individual consumer in such a way as to shield both service deliverer and the consumer from working with the complexity and the promise of the service delivery relationship. Patients may comfortably assume the choice making role when the health service they need is simple and straightforward but when this is not the case, patients are likely to want the benefit of the doctor's judgement in his or her particular case. Consider the case of HIV-treatments currently (a complex and demanding drug regime as is shown in our case study, Chapter 11): the combination drugs not only create side effects that can compromise the individual's sense of wellness and quality of life, but the manner and frequency of taking them can create major challenges for the organization of the rhythms of daily life. A treatments doctor has a complex task in preparing the patient to take the drugs, and in monitoring his or her adherence to the drug regime (see Race *et al.* 2001, 17–18). The doctor not only has to be able to 'tailor' his or her expertise to the individual patient's personality and circumstance but also to recognize that the patient may want to be guided, advised, and even directed. Here is further interview data (from Race *et al.* 2001, 14–15) where a high-HIV-caseload GP brings out the tension between the consumer model of service delivery and one that demands of the doctor the capacity to judge where to enter the fine balance of facilitating the patient's choice-making and guiding it without undermining the patient's autonomy:

It's all very nice to say that we as GPs are expected to provide the patient with informed consent and provide them with knowledge, but that is not a fair perspective ... because the patients cannot understand everything about drugs. They are looking for a GP to advise them and advice is not often based purely on fact.

Later the same GP responds to the interviewer's question in this way:

Yes, they're not just looking for knowledge; they're also looking for advice. Forever I'm getting patients saying: 'well what do you think I should do?' I present them with the information. I say well these are your options. Option one, option two, and they'll just still look at me and say, 'well what should I do?' In other words ... bugger the advice, I just want you to tell me.

The consumer model is a tempting one for doctors when they face the complexity of a patient's subjective experience and life world in how these thread through this individual's health issues and responses to these issues. If a patient presents in a relatively self-reflective way and looks like they are a practiced choice-maker, then in a post-paternalistic world, the GP will be drawn in the direction of adaptively confirming these apparent capacities of the patient rather than entering the delicate territory of probing what it is this patient may know or not know about his health and the issues it poses. When in addition a battery of technical tests for evaluating the patient's health offer along with a battery of drug treatments for health problems, the doctors is likely to draw the patient into a customized menu of diagnostic categories and treatment options where the doctor does not have to engage very deeply if at all with the inner world of the patient. This is the risk-averse and safest way of managing complexity at a time when patients are positioned as choice-making consumers even though they lack any expertise in relation to medical knowledge and where doctors, like other professionals, are permitted very little room for error.

Service deliverers have to use their professional expertise and experience to judge how best to meet an individual client's needs in what it is they have to offer. Often the exercise of professional judgement can directly match the client's expressed wants, but this does not change the fact that the exercise of professional judgement is an entirely different mode of determining the conduct of the service delivery relationship to the one that is supposed to simply follow on from and implement the will of the client. In a non-paternalistic service ethos, the service deliverer will both facilitate and listen carefully to what it is that the client says about his/her condition and what it is s/he wants to do, but when the service deliverer moves into service response, s/he is doing something other than simply realizing what it is that the consumer says s/he wants. Importantly, the service deliverer responds not just to the conscious statements of the consumer but also to his or her 'non-verbal' ways of communicating his or her sense of being in this context. Where a service deliverer works over time with the same individual client, s/he accumulates knowledge of how best to work with this person as well as maintaining a capacity to adapt to change in the client and his/her circumstances.

The consumer model of service delivery has no place for the role of professional judgement in service response. In this model, either the professional is carrying out the will of the consumer in an appropriate scientifically-informed ('evidence-based') way or the professional is deemed to be paternalistically displacing the consumer's capacity for choice. This is a profoundly impoverished conception of service delivery—one that denies the delicacy, creativity, and complexity of the service transaction as it is developed in dialogue between the service deliverer and the client. The quality of this transaction has to do with how each of these two people gives of themselves to the creation and development of their relationship.

There is an inherent asymmetrical quality of the relationship that should be valued rather than wished away. The service deliverer has both a distinctive responsibility and capacity in the relationship. The service deliverer has to take far more responsibility for ensuring that the relationship works for the client, that it is safe, civil, functionally effective, and properly bounded, than the client does. The service deliverer also has a particular service skill or capacity that the individual client needs. It is in the nature of the beast that the service deliverer knows far more than the client about this kind of relationship, its sticky and difficult aspects as well as the patterns of client response to a particular kind of care relationship. It is also in the nature of this situation that the service deliverer has or can do something the client needs, and cannot do for herself. I turn now to discussion of the service delivery relationship as intersubjective process and as a case of what Iris Young calls asymmetrical reciprocity.

Notes

1 Bigby and Fyffe (2006, 569) define institutional closure as 'the progressive reduction in the number of people with disabilities living in ... large residential facilities or the cessation of a facilities operation. In contrast,

deinstitutionalization is more complex, involving more than simply closure of institutions, requiring significant individualised support to people with intellectual disabilities as well as societal change.'

2   In Chris Clark's nuanced discussion of how community care social workers balance and seek to reconcile their respect for the self-determination of the client with their professional obligation to secure their care, he remarks of the views of the social workers he interviewed: 'Central to facilitating the client's choice was the estimate of mental soundness. Workers spoke of clients who were "unable to make a decision", not to say that it was impossible to fully ascertain the client's preferences, but meaning that the client was judged not fully cognizant of the issues and consequences because of cognitive impairment or mental health problems. Even if mental capacity were seriously impaired, workers would still hesitate to override the client's wishes. The legal safeguards of the statutory processes for compelling a client to accept help were thought to be extremely important; cutting corners by, for example, obtaining a client's purported consent for a course of action without his or her full understanding, was seen as unethical.'

6
The Inter-subjective Nature of Person-centred Service Delivery

If the client's sense of self is to be attended to and worked with in the delivery of welfare services, the service professional/worker has to be present as the self that s/he is. If the service professional/worker does not assume a lively and attentive individual presence in relation to the service client, it is unlikely that the client will feel invited to assume presence as the unique individual that s/he is in the relationship. The capacity to attend to the individuality of the client is foremost and it guides how the technical and procedural aspects of the service in question are mobilized and brought to bear on the client's situation.

In this chapter I first discuss person-centred service delivery. I then indicate the clarity of advocates of person-centred service delivery in rejecting reductionist approaches to the service user or client, approaches that treat the service user/client as a thing-like instance of a diagnostic category or some other kind of label. From there I offer a conception of what intersubjectivity in the service-delivery relationship involves and here I draw on the work of the psychoanalyst and political theorist, Jessica Benjamin, on how a genuinely intersubjective process opens up a space for what she calls thirdness. I suggest that the inherent asymmetry in the service delivery relationship cannot be wished away, but I agree with service user movements that it is meaningful to seek reciprocity and mutual recognition in this relationship. In order to reconcile the idea of mutual recognition with inherent asymmetry, I refer to the work of Iris Marion Young on 'asymmetrical reciprocity'. I briefly discuss the question of whether person-centred service delivery, an approach that is oriented to the development of the service delivery relationship as an inter-subjective one, can be used in settings where the clients are involuntary or mandated. I conclude that this is possible depending on how the wider public-moral environment impacts on the service delivery relationship, and, specifically, on whether this wider environment encourages the idea that involuntary clients (e.g. prisoners, a parent whose children will be returned to her only if she complies with court-mandated orders, people with mental illness who are subject to mandated treatment orders) have a right to be treated as 'persons'. Finally, I briefly discuss the use of self by the practitioner/ professional in the service delivery relationship. I suggest that if practitioners are to be supported in person-centred work, this is a question of how their work should be governed, a question I deal with briefly in Chapter 7.

Person-centred service delivery

I use the term 'person-centred' service delivery in this chapter for two reasons. Firstly, as argued previously (Chapter 3), when the individual is invited into relationship with others as a unique centre of subjective experience—as a self—it is because the individual enjoys the status of a person. The question of whether people get to enjoy the status of the person—to count as 'selves' in their relationships with others—is essentially a political-ethical question. This question is settled not at the level of the service delivery relationship but at the level of political society, that is, society considered in its ethical aspect and government considered in its responsibility to enable society to function ethically. The ethical nature of the service delivery relationship is essentially derivative of debates concerning personhood in its wider political-societal environment although it is fair to say also that ethical vision in service delivery has an important role in leading and contributing to these debates.

Secondly, 'person-centred' care is a term that has assumed currency especially in contemporary nursing literature, and I have found considerable congruence between the use of that term in such literature (e.g McCormack 2004; Nolan 2006; and see the similar idea of 'patient-centred care' in Miller 1997) and what it is I have in mind by an individualized approach to the delivery of welfare services that responds to the individual considered as a self.

McCormack offers a schema of person-centredness that is partially informed by Kitwood's (cit McCormack 2004, 33) definition of person-centredness as,

> ... a standing or status that is bestowed upon one human being, by others in the context of relationship and social being. It implies recognition, respect and trust.

McCormack's schema builds on this conception in elaborating what it would mean for the professional to be oriented to his/her client as a person: it would mean to understand this individual as in relationships with other persons, to understand him or her as located in a particular social world, to understand him or her as located also in place, and, finally, to welcome and appreciate their sense of self. The schema is represented in tabular form as follows (from McCormack 2004, 33):

Table 6.1 Relationship between Kitwood's definition and derived concepts of person-centredness

Concept	Link with Kitwood's definition
Being in relation	Persons exist in relationships with other persons
Being in social world	Persons are social being
Being in place	Persons have a context through which their personhood is articulated
Being with self	Being recognized, respected and trusted as a person impacts on a person's sense of self

If we recall the idea of self experience that I borrowed from Christopher Bollas (see Chapter 4), we can slightly reframe these ideas. Self experience encompasses all of these aspects: the relationship of the self to other selves who represent opportunities (and the reverse of course) for the facilitation and articulation of this individual's self experience; the relationship of the self to its situatedness in a particular historical-social-cultural modality of the world of human affairs which also represents opportunities (and the reverse) for the facilitation and articulation of self experience; the relationship of the self to its life world which is always situated in terms of place, even when it involves transposition across place as in the case of people who are immigrants, again a relationship that represents opportunities (and the reverse) for the facilitation and articulation of self experience; and finally the relationship of the self to its own experience, a relationship which depends on the capacity of the self to own and know its experience. It is the last capacity that makes it possible for an individual to have a sense of self, and, thus, provides the basis for all the other aspects of self experience. Self experience is inherently relational: there is no self prior to its articulation in experience, and it is only on the basis of such experience, that the person can be self-aware in such a way that s/he is able to engage in reflective action where choice, for example, is grounded in such self-awareness. As we saw in previous chapters (Chapters 3 and 4), no one is able to develop a capacity for self experience without the presence of others who actively facilitate self-articulation by providing a relational environment where the self feels genuinely invited to engage and safe in so doing.

This is true of any relational context, but it is especially true of welfare service delivery contexts where the self in question is not only dependent on someone else for the meeting of its needs, but where in addition the self is often highly vulnerable for reasons of acute illness, disability, poverty, stigma, or any combination of these. It is correct to recognize that the question of whether the self in these contexts is accorded the status of a person is the core ethical component of professional welfare work (remembering that I am using welfare in the broad sense to refer to all the needs of the individual considered as a self).

Very few of us are likely to go through our lifetime without finding ourselves dependent on a welfare service. For instance as Abbey *et al.* (2006, 60) point out, it is inevitable that each of us will die, and in a context where advanced medical care is available, it is likely that many of us will die relatively slowly, and at an advanced old age, thus suggesting a period of considerable dependence on formal and informal caregivers. It is therefore important that there is a public appreciation on the part of both citizens and government that welfare work has a vital role to play in whether we get to enjoy the status of the person. Positively speaking, if such work supports and facilitates our individual personhood, it can do much to enhance our personhood and sense of self; by the same token, such work can also be of destructive impact on our personhood and sense of self precisely because, at the time of our dependence on welfare work, we are subject to others who have the power to withhold, or damage, our status as a person.

Of course, as many authors (Hoggett 2000, Chapter 9; Cooper and Lousada 2005, 42–44) point out, a major barrier to a popular-public understanding of the crucial significance of welfare work to personhood is fear of dependence, vulnerability and abjection. Abbey *et al.* (2006, 60) in discussing the place of palliative care in long-term care at this point of time cite another set of authors who propose considerable popular resistance to acceptance of the inevitability of death:

> Despite polls reporting a widespread public pragmatism about death and dying ('I would never want to be a vegetable', 'When my time comes I do not want to be kept alive artificially'), when clinicians do try to discuss treatment abatement with patients and families, they often meet disbelief, even hostility. Clearly, polls reflect public attitudes as distinct from personal situations. In personal health care encounters, the idea that cure is improbable or impossible, or that

continued life support is inappropriate or unkind, is unacceptable to many families. The wider problem here is that an acknowledgment of the inevitability of death and preparation for it, have largely lost their place in our culture.

Such lack of acknowledgment also means an inability of the public to accept that resource scarcity must assume a place in discussions of how viable it is to use technological and pharmacological artifice to keep people alive when otherwise they would die.

It is because the personhood of the welfare service user is at risk in the service delivery relationship that welfare service user movements have been so antagonistic to the power of the professional in the service delivery relationship. They have sought ways of enhancing the power of the service user in order to counter the power of the professional with the important aim of making the relationship more symmetrical. There can be no doubt of the historical importance of the rhetoric of welfare service user empowerment, for it has clearly contributed to the evolution of a more refined and post-paternalistic professional conception of person-centred care; but it is a category error to think that the relationship between client and professional can be reframed so as to avoid the asymmetry that arises from the professional being able to offer something that the client needs. As I argued in Chapter 5, this category error has translated into the consumption model of the service delivery relationship where the service client is repositioned as a consumer whose will is to be served by the professional/service worker. This model comes at considerable cost because it displaces the autonomy of the professional worker and of the profession that shapes the ethos and technical knowledge base of such work. Neither of these can be adequately valued because instead of being regarded as a living, creative, and active contribution to making the personhood of individuals possible—to enabling their self-preservation (see the discussion of the right to self-preservation as the core human right in Chapter 3)—the individual professional, and his/her profession are simply regarded as technical means of realizing the will of the individual consumer or of government positioned as the purchaser of services in a quasi-(service)market. To put this slightly differently: when professional work is situated within the causality of a means-end relationship directed by a sovereign will, it is essentially deprived of its enlivening features and turned into the inanimate nature of a technical process that is judged in relation to equally inanimate formal performance standards and measures.

Nevertheless, it is meaningful to attempt to conceive and practice an asymmetrical relationship so that it is open to an inter-subjective reciprocity. I shall discuss this further shortly.

Rejection of reductionist and reified conceptions of the service user

It is of note that a good deal of contemporary writing from professionals about how to conceive their work so that it attends to the needs of the self of those they work with is so clear about what it means to work with the individual as a person, or in Hegelian language, as a subject of right. In such writing we find a clear rejection of models of service delivery that view the individual in terms of a diagnostic category or through the grid of a formal set of procedures that are to be applied to people in this particular category.

Here is Brendan McCormack, a professor of nursing research, on this point in relation to gerontological nursing:

> The history of nursing suggests that [older people] ... were not treated as persons, particularly in large institutions, but instead conformed to rigid rules and boundaries that served the needs of the organization more than the older person.

> But is there an *a priori* set of characteristics that define a person? It is conceivable to hold a concept of persons based on physical and psychological characteristics. Indeed, reductionist approaches to research would be an example of how often we do this. Reductionist models don't adopt a whole-person approach, but instead attempt to study particular characteristics, behaviours, responses, emotions for example, and then relate these to general features of (say) ageing processes or functional ability. In clinical practice, a common example of this is the making of judgements about an older person's competence to be involved in decision-making or ability to cope with particular levels of care provision on the basis of a single assessment (e.g. minimental health test). This narrow perspective of persons has the potential for individuals not to be treated as persons and indeed to be reduced to a 'thing' (McCormack 2004, 32).

Here is another example of such clarity concerning the importance of not viewing an individual as the instantiation of a category of being that is already known about in relation to an expert-based classification. People with mental illness have been and still are amongst those most vulnerable to expert-driven reification of their being. Here is Suzanne Shuda, a clinical psychologist working in South Africa, in a piece of writing co-authored with Anna, someone who has had multiple admissions to psychiatric hospitals since she was 17 in 1976, and who was suicidal at the time she came to work with Suzanne:

> To continue to move away from the fixed representation of people's experience has been an ongoing professional and personal challenge for me. For instance, reading about people's lives, as professionally or clinically documented by another writer, is intolerable to me at the moment. It seems of vital importance that the world somehow takes note of how we all become deadened by dominant discourses about clinical practices. If writing will not allow the voice of the person to be present in its raw form, how will we address the issue of wanting to disengage from life? My attempt to keep despair and hopelessness at bay is simply to try to listen carefully to each word (Suzanne Shuda and Just Anna 2007, 88).

Anna writes eloquently about her experience in hospital and, for reasons she explains, it is clear that her hospital file has come to assume a menacing presence in her life:

> One needs a lot of time to recover from the shock of being in a hospital. I know what it is like to be in those wards. I know I will feel even worse if I have to go back. I have slit my wrists, tried to suffocate myself, and hang myself. I once tried to strangle myself with a surgical glove. I remember ill people and buckets of urine. I remember trying to drink water out of a toilet. I once ran away out of a locked ward. I squeezed out through a broken window and went to the police. I was taken back the next day. We were treated like cattle. I was the only white person and there was an inverse racism going on. People were often beaten up. I used to take a rock and hit myself on the head. I felt so utterly worthless. One of the night nurses told me that there were many terrible things written in my file that they all knew about. I am even scared to think of it now. I never felt that I was taken seriously. I was observed, judged and written off. I stayed in hospital because my family would not have me back home (Suzanne Shuda and Just Anna 2007, 91).

Anna continues this segment of her writing and says simply, 'I would like people to know that people in hospital have feelings whether they are psychotic or not' (Suzanne Shuda and Just Anna 2007, 91).

When Anna begins to work with Suzanne, she (Anna) has begun to find ways of staying out of hospital, and she experiences in her talking to Suzanne that, as reflected back to her by a team working with Suzanne, 'this has made your experiences real because she listens and has given you words to hold onto (Suzanne Shuda and Just Anna 2007, 92)'. Suzanne and Anna decide 'it would be valuable for Anna to have access to the dreaded hospital file' (Suzanne Shuda and Just Anna 2007, 93). With the new South African constitution, it was now possible to have access to a copy of the file. The file turned out to be 100 pages with admissions only going back to 1994, while Anna's first admission had been in 1976. Here is Suzanne on Anna's response as they together began reading the file:

> Anna remembered three files being wheeled in on a trolley for case discussions, a history hard to leave behind her, following her into every new admission, being used as an important reference point in every discussion with or about her. Here it was, safely in her hands … Anna's initial apprehension gave way to outrage. We read faster and faster and then just jumped forward through the entries, catching diagnoses and descriptions of her behaviour here and there. At times Anna spoke of events and her memories of them. Suddenly Anna sat back, laughed and said: 'The file says nothing. *Nothing* about who I am or of what has happened to me. They never knew who I was, what I thought or what I felt. They knew nothing. They are just their words. I am somebody else.' Anna was amazed and relieved from the idea that '*the file*' had had such importance in her life (Suzanne Shuda and Just Anna 2007, 94, emphases in the original).

Anna has clearly portrayed a situation in which, in hospital, she was not positioned as a person but as a slave in the sense discussed in Chapter 3. There I introduced the idea of slavery in political theory as meaning the subjection of an individual to the arbitrary will of another; this is a relationship of domination, one where the person who is dominated cannot express their sense of self for fear of risking the dominator's payback or, even if she does, she is utterly disregarded. Anna's combination of disbelief and relief that her file turned out to contain nothing in which she could recognize herself mirrors Joanna Penglase's discovery, regarding the personal records of state wards in Australia, that these contained nothing 'personal'. Speaking of the present (Penglase 2005, 323), she says:

[Ex] State wards, from any state, have a reasonable, although not guaranteed, chance of getting their personal files from the Departments involved [if they have not been destroyed as is the case with some of these agencies]. If there were problems in their care history, it may even be a substantial file, but it will still be impersonal and often judgemental. It will be 'personal' only in the sense that it has their name on it: it will not be a record of their development through childhood, except in terms of how the authorities regarded them—terms such as 'high grade mental defective', 'slow but not mentally retarded', 'backward', 'difficult', 'insubordinate' and so on.

Intersubjectivity in the service delivery relationship

Anna found Suzanne through the help of a friend; and she began working with Suzanne at a very low point in her life when she had just been discharged from a mental hospital. Anna says of the point at which she began to work with Suzanne:

[She] reached out to me and slowly extracted a tiny splinter of hope. With faith she gave me goals each week that got me to believe that the extreme effort required would be of worthwhile consequence (Suzanne Shuda and Just Anna 2007, 89).

After working together for five years, Anna had learned to live with her illness (bipolar disorder) and had found a place in the world that was satisfying to her and to others. Suzanne comments:

Anna is currently living in Cape Town with her mother and is a sought-after caretaker of young and old. She has a dog called Daisy who was abandoned and who has become attached, loyal, playful and friendly. Anna and Daisy love to go on walks. She continues to write poetry and make cards ... We still meet once a fortnight to talk about her life and to write (see Suzanne Shuda and Just Anna 2007, 97–98)

What Anna was able to do with Suzanne was to co-create an intersubjective process wherein each felt recognized by the other as well as reciprocally invited to creatively contribute to making this relationship generative for Anna's growth and healing. Anna experienced for the first time a professional's attention, care, and 'holding' (in the sense of Winnicott's term) that enabled her sense of self to be gathered, articulated, and then made available for her to think about. We can see in these short excerpts I have taken from this piece of co-writing by Suzanne and Anna that each of these two people— Suzanne in a professional capacity; Anna in a client capacity—felt sufficient trust in the other to be free to actively give of their self to the building and development of their relationship. Anna did not feel judged by Suzanne, or treated by Suzanne as a thing—as, simply, the individual exemplification of her class of mental disorder. Instead, Anna felt invited to come alive as a person in relating to Suzanne, and in this process of coming alive, Anna could develop her own inner strength, determination to change her life, and to engage creatively with the challenge of living.

Jessica Benjamin (2004, 5), an object relations psychoanalyst who has rich background in Hegelian social and political theory, offers a clear and useful definition of inter-subjectivity:

> ... a relation in which each person experiences the other as a 'like subject,' another mind who can be 'felt with,' yet has a distinct, separate centre of feeling and perception. The antecedents of my perspective on intersubjectivity lie on the one hand with Hegel ... and on the other with the developmentally oriented thinkers Winnicott and Stern—quite different in their own ways—who try to specify the process by which we become able to grasp the other as having a separate yet similar mind.

It is so easy for professionals to treat people, especially people who live with cognitive impairment of some kind, as simply thing-like instantiations of their diagnostic label. Yet it is so clear that it makes all the difference in the world to these individuals when they are invited to participate in an inter-subjective relationship with welfare workers. If Anna's story were not enough, here are two other examples. In a study of 16 self-advocates with intellectual disability in Australia, Shaddock *et al.* (1993, 47–49) found that these individuals insisted on three themes: firstly, people with disabilities are people first, not service users; secondly, 'independence should not be made the most important goal for people with intellectual disabilities—relationships are more important'; and, thirdly, that the involvement between them and the service provider is all important. On this last theme, the participants in the study 'emphasised [the importance of service workers] listening to all forms of communicative behaviour, such as taking time to read communication boards, or interpret a person's gestures or facial expressions. One participant noted that challenging behaviour was a form of communication and should be responded to as such.' In this last point we can see an insistence on the service delivery relationship as an inter-subjective one. The second example concerns people living with dementia. Louise Nolan (2006, 209) cites other colleagues working in gerontological nursing as proposing that 'preservation of personhood is central to quality dementia care', and that 'inter-subjectivity between nurse and person' is the key to such care. She cites research which shows that an inter-subjective relationship of this kind, where the nurse takes the time to build a relationship with the older person and to get to know him or her, as well as his or her relatives/carers, promotes lucidity while 'impersonal care reduces the chances of persons with dementia using latent capabilities' (Nolan 2006, 212). She concludes: 'The findings suggest that nurses in an acute care setting consider the lives of persons with dementia meaningful and that lucidity and communication are possible through participatory caring (Nolan 2006, 213).' Each of us, I would suggest, finds it easier to be lucid and communicative if we are invited to share space with another person who extends to us not just welcome but also non-judgemental and attentive recognition.

Jessica Benjamin (2004, 6) suggests that inter-subjectivity is operative when we are able to experience the other as both 'a separate and yet connected being with whom we are acting reciprocally'. In this inter-subjective process of relating, she argues, the individuals concerned create 'thirdness'. By this she means that these individuals are not locked into a dyadic pattern of complementarity that is based either in mutual identification (fusion) or in each feeling that s/he has either to submit to or resist the other's demand (see Benjamin 2004, 9–10). In a complementary structure of the relationship, 'dependency becomes coercive', and reactivity is the modality of the response of each to the other. It is a relationship characterized by impasse rather than by an openness to creative exploration together of possibilities: 'each person feels done to, and not like an agent helping to shape a co-created reality' (Benjamin 2004, 9). The thirdness refers to the space that opens up in a genuinely co-created reality, a space for the expression of individual differences, a space for the mutual discovery of hitherto unknown possibilities of communication and interaction, and a relational space that makes inner space in each participant possible. Thirdness stands for both an ethical orientation to recognition of each other's personhood, and for the subjective capacity to learn how to engage in practicing such an orientation. The achievement of thirdness is always fragile and liable to breakdown, especially if the practitioner begins to judge herself for some reason, an attitude to self that must affect her capacity to engage non-judgementally and in a listening mode with the client.

Benjamin suggests there is an inherent tendency for inter-subjectivity to break down into complementarity, but if the psycho-analyst is able to recognize when this occurs, a process in which she must have been collusive, then she is able to recover 'the intersubjective view' (Benjamin 2004, 29), and open up the space of inter-subjectivity again:

> In effect, we tell ourselves, whatever we have done that has gotten us into the position of being in the wrong is not so horribly shameful that we cannot own it. It stops being submission to the patient's reality because, as we free ourselves from shame and blame, the patient's accusation no longer persecutes us, and hence, we are no longer in the grip of helplessness. It is no longer a matter of which person is sane, right, health, knows best, or the like, and if the analyst is able to acknowledge the patient's suffering without stepping into the position of badness, then the intersubjective space of thirdness is restored. My point is that this step out of helplessness [the complementarity position of 'coerced dependency'] usually involves more than an internal process; it involves direct or transitionally framed ... communication about one's own reactivity, misattunement, or misunderstanding. *By making a claim on the potential space of thirdness, we call upon it, and so call it into being* (Benjamin 2004, 33, emphases added).

Dependency, then, does not have to be coercive; it can be generative, and congruent with an inter-subjective process that facilitates the personhood of each individual in the relationship. Just as the parent with the child has responsibility for ensuring the relationship is open rather than closed, inter-subjective rather than complementary, so too does the professional have such responsibility in regard to the service delivery relationship. Here is a description from the point of view of the patient of how her breast cancer nurse specialist interacted with her on doing a biopsy. In it can be seen how this nurse specialist interacts with the patient—herself a nurse-researcher and teacher who thus has the observational skills to offer such a description—in such a way as to provide containment for the patient's emotional experience as well as to open up this space of inter-subjectivity that Benjamin talks of:

> E's skill and respect for me as a patient were evident in a number of ways, on this occasion and on all succeeding occasions. I told her I was scared. I would have told anyone but she made it easy to say to her and her reaction, which was minimal, did not make me feel foolish. Her behaviour made it entirely clear that she had under-stood my terror and was reacting accordingly. E knew I was an academic before she met me, so her conversation during the biopsy, clearly designed to distract me, utilised that knowledge. She told me about her Masters degree and the essay she stayed up all night word processing and which had got lost. The topic was familiar enough to hold my attention and to remind me of situations in which I was a competent 'grown up' person; thus boosting my self-esteem and confidence. I nearly passed out at one point. Her skill in dealing with that was very evident—position, comfort, maintaining the cir-cumstances which allowed the biopsy to continue; afterwards a glass of really cold water, keeping someone with me when she had to go. And everything done in a way which allowed me to maintain my dignity (Niven and Scott 2003, 205).

Asymmetrical reciprocity in the service-delivery relationship

As I have said, it is understandable that service user movements have sought to bring about reciprocity within the relationship between service deliverer and client. However, generally speaking, they have done this within the orientation of what Benjamin calls complemen-tarity. They have viewed the relationship as essentially a dyadic one structured by a power struggle over whose will is to prevail: is one to 'do' or to be 'done to'? Not only does a complementary structure fore-close a space for inter-subjective process but it essentially makes it difficult if not impossible for the professional worker in the relation-ship to assume responsibility, or at least more responsibility than the service user, for orienting the relationship to reciprocal recognition of separate though connected persons within what is a shared project of some kind.

The complementary structuring of a relationship relates to what Iris Young calls 'symmetrical reciprocity'. With a desire for symmetrical reciprocity, the subject feels both entitled and able to put herself in the other's shoes. Such a desire is essentially one of the subject's identification with the other, and it is identification that closes the intersubjective space of thirdness. Once identification is operative, the other either has to comply with the subject's projection or to dumbly resist it.

When Iris Young offers the idea of 'asymmetrical reciprocity', then, she does this in context of a critique of the idea of symmetrical reciprocity, 'the claim that moral respect requires that each of us should take the perspective of all the others in making our moral judgments' for three reasons. First, 'the idea of symmetry' 'obscures the difference and particularity of the other position (Young 1997, 44)'. She argues that even when individuals 'find their relations defined by similarly socially structured differences of gender, race, class, nation, or religion, individuals usually also find many ways in which they are strange to one another (Young 1997, 45)'. Congruent with the idea of self experience that I have offered, Young proposes that 'individuals bring different life histories, emotional habits, and life plans to relationships, which make their positions irreversible'. Young (1997, 45) argues further that the idea of symmetrical reciprocity 'closes off the creative exchange these differences might produce with one another'. Here, in effect, Young is arguing against the dyadic structure of mutual identification in favour of what Benjamin calls thirdness, an openness to inter-subjective space. Second, Young (1997, 44) argues that 'it is ontologically impossible for people in one social position to adopt the perspective of those in the social positions with which they are related in social structures and interaction'. She uses the example of mother and daughter, proposing that while these two individuals share 'social positions of gender, race, class' etc, there is an inherent asymmetry of age and generation; but not only that, 'their relation is itself internally constituted by the asymmetry of positioning between them and the desires and projections that produces' (Young 1997, 47). Third, Young argues that the idea that 'moral respect involves taking the other' person's point of view can have 'politically undesirable consequences' (Young 1997, 44). Essentially, it is no longer necessary to listen to the other with awareness that one does not know the other and cannot know the other except through the opening that listening to the other's communication creates.

Young, then, firmly holds onto the idea that the perspectives of subjects are irreducibly asymmetrical. She suggests this is so in two important ways. First, each subject has its own history, a temporality, that lends a unique depth to his or her perspective, most of which never surfaces in communication with another: 'Each person brings to a communication situation the particular experiences, assumptions, meanings, symbolic associations, and so on, that emerge from a particular history, most of which lies as background to the communicating situation (Young 1997, 51).' Secondly, 'asymmetry refers also to the specificity of *position*' (Young 1997, 51)'. Young proposes that 'each social position is structured by the configuration among positions': 'If we recognize that subject positions and perspectives are multiply structured in relation to many other positions ... the specificity and irreversibility of each location is more obvious.' In the case of the subject positions of service professional and service client/user, these will be always highly specific in terms of type of welfare service, organizational setting, and the policy-jurisdictional context of the service. Each of these two subject positions is aligned quite differently in relation to other subject positions: those for example of organizational management, the user's friends and informal carers, policy makers, and so on.

Young further develops her idea of asymmetrical reciprocity in the ideas of gift-giving, communication and wonder. She suggests that symmetrical equivalence in gift-giving is morally inappropriate; it closes rather than opens up the relationship. She suggests that:

> The gift is a unique offering. The only proper response is acceptance. The relation of offering and acceptance is asymmetrical; I do not return, I accept. If later I give you a gift, it is a new offering, with its own asymmetry (Young 1997, 54).

Secondly, the temporal separation of moments of gift-giving is central to how this kind of exchange contributes to the building of a relationship that extends into the future. Here Young cites Irigaray in suggesting 'the gift gives time': 'It demands time, the thing, but it demands a delimited time, neither an instant nor an infinite time, but a time determined by a term, in other words, a rhythm, a cadence' (Young 1997, 54–55). Here Young comes close to Benjamin's discussion of how rhythms of mutual accommodation in human interaction 'help constitute the capacity for thirdness': 'rhythmicity may be seen as model principle underlying the creation of shared patterns' (Benjamin 2004, 17). It is in the nature of mutual accommodation for one's response to the action of the other to create a new temporal interval which, in turn, invites a new response of accommodation from the other.

Communication, Young, suggests also functions similarly: the listener's response to the speaker open up another turn in the creation of a dynamic process of meaning that is shared at least in a good enough way and of meaning that fails to be shared (these are my words rather than Young's). It is again an inherently asymmetrical process. Young (1997, 55–56) stresses the importance of the listener's orientation as being one of not knowing what it is the other is going to communicate, nor of knowing what it means exactly without seeking further information. This is where wonder comes in for Young: 'without also a moment of wonder, of openness to the newness and mystery of the other person, the creative energy of desire dissolves into indifference (Young 2004, 56)'.

Involuntary or mandated clients

The ethical conception of the service delivery relationship in terms of intersubjective process applies independently of whether the clients concerned are voluntary or involuntary (mandated). Involuntary clients include people who have been charged with a crime and are situated somewhere in the corrections system as well as people who are subject to compliance with certain officially prescribed conditions if they are to receive income support, treatment, to have their children returned to them, to be able to see their partner, or to have access to some other aspect of normal civil standing.

The question in contexts where people are subject to the force of the state turns on the rationale for the use of such force. If it is designed simply to control people then the issue of service delivery does not arise. But if the rationale for the use of force, at least in part, is to provide an intervention designed to assist the individual in achieving skills and subjective capacity that enable him or her to meet his or her adult responsibilities in a lawful, peaceful, and effective way then it makes sense to dovetail the imposition of restraining conditions with service facilitation of the individual's development of such skills and subjective capacity. This is how Sue Vardon (former director-general of the South Australian Department for Correctional Services who is discussed further in the case study, Chapter 13) is thinking when she defends the proposition that prisoners are clients too. She argues: 'the important issue is that offenders are recognised as the principal recipients of the [correctional system] agency and should be responded to with appropriate individual plans based on the belief that intervention can be more constructive than it is presently, and that the whole organisation has a role to change and improve to achieve this goal (Vardon 1997, 128)'. She is aware that some individuals in prison will not want to take advantage of such opportunities, but comments: 'Surprisingly many do want to change and take the opportunities to learn' an alternative way than that of crime to realize their personal goals.

Peter De Jong and Insoo Kim Berg (2001) offer the practice of 'solution-focused interviewing' as a way of engaging involuntary and mandated clients. This is a practice focused on enabling the client to 'be their own authority on what they want changed in their lives and how to make these changes happen (De Jong and Berg 2001, 363)'. Without identifying with the client, or taking his or her side against the system, the practitioner respects the client's sense of what is happening and why, focuses on the client's past successes and strengths, and facilitates the client working through what it is that s/he needs to do in order to achieve his or her goals. They discuss at length, providing relevant interview transcription material, the case of 'Diana', a mother who has been incarcerated, and whose children have been put in foster care. She has to meet certain requirements—employment, attendance at AA meetings, etc.—before her children can be returned to her. It is clear from the transcribed interview material where Diana and the practitioner are talking together, that the practitioner Berg's approach is not unlike that of Suzanne Shuda in working with Anna (discussed above). Berg begins by getting to know Diana and in this process Berg assumes what these authors call a 'not knowing' role:

> ... unlike other approaches in which practitioners turn next to reviewing information already in the case record with which mandated clients often take issue [remember how Anna felt about her hospital file], Berg remained not knowing and asked how it was that the court came to send Diana to this agency. She also asked what the court wanted to be different as a result of her contact with the agency and what Diana's view was about the court and agency's expectations for her. In addition to keeping Diana in the role of expert, these questions also differentiated Berg from the court and agency with their expectations for Diana. This differentiation set the stage for Berg and Diana to co-construct a way to cooperate regarding what Diana wanted to do about the circumstances she faced in her mandated situation (De Jong and Berg 2001, 364).

Another significant point of difference with established approaches, where the practitioner assumes the voice of control, in telling the client what she has to do to satisfy the mandating conditions, in this case Berg, the practitioner, asks Diana, 'What needs to come out of this, so that you can say, okay, this was not my idea, but hey, this turned out to be good for me?' Diana takes up this invitation to differentiate between what the mandating authority requires of her, and what she thinks of these requirements. She responds by saying she has already done 7/8 of the things on her contract, but that she refuses to sign the contract because she disagrees with what it says. In expressing her disagreement, she is indicating her own judgement as to what she needs to do in order to get her life in order in order to resume parenting. Here is the interview passage concerned:

> *Diana*: They state that I need to go to a domestic violence counselling now. Which I disagree with. I have had domestic violence with the father of my two daughters, severe violence—four years of it. I lived through it. I overcame it. I got out of it. I did not have another episode of physical violence until a year ago. I feel I do not need it. They also mandated me ... I had to go to AA and I had to get slips signed to show proof. And the worker states she needs this ... For the first six months that I was with the agency, I was going on my own. I do drink excessively. I'm what you call a problem drinker. ... My worker and myself we have a good rapport. But we do hit heads. ... as I told her, I feel I don't have to show her diddly-squat ... And as I told her, I don't mind going to AA. I like AA ... It's a lot of helpful things I learn in there. But I don't feel I have to prove it.
> *Berg*: That's the part you disagree with. Having to prove yourself.
> *Diana*: Right. And then she wants to meet with my sponsor. And everyone knows who knows anything about AA, it's an anonymous program ...

Berg does not ask Diana to simply comply on rational-pragmatic grounds with the requirements so she can get her boys back, knowing that for Diana, 'my boys mean everything to me'. Rather Berg respects Diana's position, and 'remains not knowing and impartial about what Diana should do in her situation' (De Jong and Berg 2001, 368), while continuing to facilitate Diana's own ideas for solutions. De Jong and Berg (2001, 371) comment of the end of the session with Diana:

It is clear from her comments that Diana was struggling and suffering in her current circumstances. She was at an impasse with the agency, feeling as though she could not contractually agree to its requirements without unacceptably compromising herself. Again, it can be imagined that Berg might be tempted to say: 'Yes, I hear what you said, but ...' and turn to interventions of confrontation and education blended with empathy. To do so, however, would be to fail to listen carefully to Diana, to disrespect her current constructions, and to undermine her responsibility for what to do next. One solution-focused option at this point is to affirm that Diana is struggling and ask questions about how she is managing to cope in such difficult circumstances ... Berg did this and Diana responded with details about how she was drawing on God, friends, and her love for her children to keep herself going. The use of coping questions is consistent with a strengths approach ... which assumes that even under the harshest of conditions clients are taking actions on their own behalf by drawing on their competencies (De Jong and Berg 2001, 371).

De Jong and Berg (2001, 371) are alert to the dynamic and generative character of intersubjective process, aware that the client will keep on processing after the session has finished: 'Experience has taught us that client constructions are always in process and that the not-knowing questions asked during the interview continue to be processed by the client after the client leaves the sessions.'

Working with involuntary/mandated clients in a way that opens up the relationship to intersubjective process presupposes a differentiation of role between the agent who imposes the constraint on the client and the conditions attached to the client's freedom from such constraint, and the agent(s) who work with the client in the context of such constraint. It is possible to engage the involuntary/mandated client in person-centred service delivery if the wider policy and political environment does not pre-empt this. Practitioner vision of what can and should be done in these contexts needs to inform wider policy and public debate. At the same time those responsible for sentencing offenders, and for prescribing conditions other clients have to meet if they are to be released from some kind of constraint, need to know how their judgements impact on people. A senior manager in an Australian State corrections system told us (this project's research team):

There is no system ... to get the judiciary ... to understand the impact of their behaviour. ...The judges seem to be blissfully unaware of the impact of what they do; ... they're actually the ones who are ... making the decision about when someone will come to gaol, when they'll leave, and what type of things they might expect someone to do during that time. In any situation ... that I've brought the judges face to face with the offenders, which happens ... rarely ... it's been quite extraordinary. ... I had an event recently with the Judicial Commission [in a specific State] where we try and educate them about the impact of their behaviour ... I brought a young Aboriginal woman to meet them, who was in custody, and I had the extremely punitive judge who had just sentenced someone to ... 45 years in relation to a rape charge, and I had [name of a progressive Aboriginal magistrate] and I was there like that with all those divergent views, and they all had an incredible impact of seeing this person ... They ... made all these statements to her, like saying ... you have a drinking problem, and she spoke about the type of work that she'd done, and all the deaths that had happened to her in the space of about a year, all ... immediate family. And they were completely overcome and a number of them wrote to me at the end, they all came personally and thanked her for this type of opportunity. ... this person wasn't representative of anyone other than herself. In other words, she wasn't the typical Aboriginal woman or anything ...

Use of self on the part of the professional

The professional/practitioner's capacity to attend respectfully and creatively to the reality of the client's sense of self demands of the former not just a professional set of skills but also a practice of self-reflection and self-knowledge that enables him or her to know when s/he is contributing to opening up or closing down intersubjective process. Good professionals/ practitioners who are able to sustain their work will be those who know how to look after and to attend to their own sense of self. A highly stressed, overworked and inadequately supported professional/practitioner is likely to find it hard to work in this way or to sustain working in this way. In addition, the professional/practitioner who works in this way is as Niven and Scott (2003, 206) point out, exposed to his/her own as well as to the client's/patient's distress. For this reason it is important that the agency environment of the professional/practice provide supervision and peer support that enables him/her to contain his/her feelings.

The policy environment of intersubjective process in service delivery

If service delivery is to be person-centred, professionals must feel that they have the trust and support of the policy environment that frames their work. As Cooper and Lousada (2005, 46) put it, there needs to be a 'protected space for the internal world of welfare' where professionals can work with service clients/users in building the kind of relationship that sustains intersubjective process. They explain what it is they mean by the 'internal world' of welfare:

> In welfare this is, or should be, a place where sensitive, private, complex, ambiguous, and perhaps shameful matters are negotiated, thought about, and acted upon. Obviously, this should be in a way that relates to the 'external world' of policy, procedure, service organization, and so on, but it should not be dominated or intruded upon by this world more than is absolutely necessary. It is possible to think about the conception and implementation of welfare in this way, from the most mundane and local of transactions through to how we understand the ultimate aims of grand policy reforms and transformation of structure. Looked at this way, the object of welfare is to make available resources (education, mental health services, fostering, well woman clinics, housing stock, and so on) with which people can engage in a manner that enables them to effect transformation in their circumstances, because the impact of their needs and demands is taken in, recognized, metabolized and respected (Cooper and Lousada 2005, 46).

I have argued that, as far as welfare is concerned, it is the design and practice of professionally oriented service delivery that can make the difference as to whether individuals are able to effectively enjoy the status of a person or not. The professions that contribute to welfare so understood have a core public mission. As I argued in Chapter 2, this mission is not new even though its contemporary iteration is much more adequate to an intersubjective ethic of personhood. It is important that a conception of government as one that facilitates the public mission of the welfare professions be developed and also become a central subject of public discussion and debate. I turn to a brief discussion of such a conception of government in the next chapter.

7
Governing Welfare Services

The inner world of welfare services mirrors the inner world of the society that comes under the jurisdiction of contemporary democratic constitutional government. Both are extraordinarily complex: their internal segmentation into distinct spheres of activity is highly elaborated; the question of authority has become far more complex in a setting where hierarchy has to be flexibly engaged and negotiated with those who are subject to it; organizational boundaries have become more porous and fluid and horizontal networks now complement if not supplant vertical structures of integration; and, with all this, people expect to find subjective meaning in their relationships and to be able to express their sense of self in them.

Reduction of complexity is likely to be the first thing any decision maker will attempt to achieve in considering the task of governing such a world, whether it is the world of welfare services or that of society at large. There are, however, different ways of achieving the reduction of complexity, and there are two alternate frameworks for going about so doing. The first of these frameworks is oriented in terms of control supplemented by delegation to the authority of private property. The second of these frameworks is oriented in terms of the facilitation of ground-level stakeholder cooperation in learning how to respond creatively and effectively to challenges for action.

Government control supplemented by delegation to the authority of private property

In this framework, government maintains control over a residual set of welfare functions targeted essentially to people who for various reasons are unable to achieve market-based self-reliance. The objective of such control is essentially to ensure that the existence of these people does not constitute too great a social nuisance or cost for those who fit the model of normal personhood: the self-reliant individual with his or her dependants. In a society oriented to a more egalitarian communitarian conception of citizenship—Australia for example as distinct from the United States—the control function of government extends also to the public funding of services for the deserving poor (home care for old age pensioners for example) and to some minimal level of universal health care. As the direct funder of welfare services such as a public hospital system for example, on the control approach, government emphasizes cost-containment, and adopts a method of controlling the hospital sector in order to achieve this goal.

Beyond the sphere of welfare services for which government continues to have direct responsibility as the funding agency, government creates institutional incentives to privatize all other welfare services. Here the economists' conception of the elegance of the market economy as a way of managing complexity prevails. It is assumed that the multiplicity and variety of consumer preferences will be matched by service development; that people will get what they are willing to pay for; and that for-profit providers competing with one another will be forced to innovate and achieve greater cost-effectiveness in order to stay in business. From the point of view of individualization in the delivery of welfare services, the great advantage of this approach is that people who need services are positioned as private agents who can realize their preferences (their will) in finding the right service for them.

The primary difficulties with this approach are two-fold, each of them matching the two components of the model: a method of governing that is control-focused; and a reliance on market principles. The method of governing that is control-focused, inevitably, imposes a top-down policy approach that is conceived at considerable distance from ground-level complexities. In the control orientation, policy is easily captured by the dual imperative of political pandering to the electorate, on the one hand, and a narrow as well as generic idea of cost containment on the other. Policy development in this framework is not informed by a substantive orientation to the sphere of welfare services in question where the policy makers seek to learn how best to govern this sphere in its specific requirements of government: responding for example to the real costs of service provision, to the inevitable difference of perspective of the different stakeholders in this field of service provision (e.g. victim groups, sentencing judges, prison management and officers, and prisoners in the field of correctional services), and considering long-term issues of sustainability of this area of service provision as these implicate workforce planning, managing the variables that affect numbers of people in prison which, in turn, impacts on the costs of this sector, the impact of re-offending on the community, and so on.

The other problem that arises in regard to reliance on market solutions concerns the intersubjective nature of welfare services (discussed in the previous chapter). A service response that fits the sense of self of an individual in context of his or her life world is what makes the difference to whether this individual's needs are met or not. Welfare services are irreducible to the simplicity of the consumption model associated with the market economy, a model that is predicated on a private property owner purchasing a thing, where possession of the thing actualizes the will of the individual consumer. Many wealthy consumers, no doubt, regard welfare services as things that they can purchase, and consider it appropriate that once they have paid someone to give them a welfare service it makes sense for them, the consumer, to direct this employee in how s/he does this work. However, as I have argued in Chapter 5, the consumer model of service delivery is not adequate to the nature of welfare services. Firstly, it cannot be assumed that the consciously expressed desire (will) of the consumer is in fact the only or even the best expression of their needs for a welfare service. As Niven and Scott (2003, 202) say of the nursing context, 'when people are at their most vulnerable, they are often least able to identify, or even to express, their need—beyond the completely obvious'. Secondly, a service that is responsive to the sense of self of the individual who needs the service has to be provided by a trained worker. This is someone who maintains standards of care, feels accountable to an impartial observer of this care relationship, and is personally committed to a public ethic of care. This is a professionalism that has to be accorded its own autonomy, relative of course to the other stakeholders in a public economy of welfare services. However in a private welfare service market, professionalism cannot be accorded even this relative autonomy in the face of the business imperative of staying competitive. Professionalism in such a setting is externally directed by a purpose that is foreign to its nature.

Where welfare services are situated within a private service market economy, their relative quality will reflect the class or 'market' standing (wealth) of those who need them. Such services will divide into high end and low end service sectors. However, as I have suggested already, even the high end service sector, while replete with all that money can buy, will not be able to provide what money cannot buy: a public service ethic that is oriented to reflective practice, ongoing learning and professional training, and a passionate commitment to the provision of service that makes a real difference to people considered as persons. Furthermore a private service market corrupts the professionals who are positioned in such a market. Instead of looking to a career structure that enables them to engage deeply, continuously and in a way that accumulates learning and experience in a professional service ethic, they displace the primacy of this band of motivation by being forced to consider their relative earnings as a measure of professional success. Once this set of incentives are in play, all aspects of a professional career are viewed in terms of investment opportunities and costs; thus the costs of professional training and education are viewed as a private investment enabling the individual a market advantage s/he would not otherwise have, and also promoting the determination to recoup these costs once the individual is able to sell his or her services in the marketplace.

Of course, the workers in a private service market will also divide into a minority of those who can command relatively good levels of pay for their services, and a growing majority of poorly paid and under-valued workers whose work conditions offer them very little protection, security, or safety. Workers will stay in such jobs only as long as there is no good alternative. There is no space or incentive for them to engage in training and learning associated with their work. Serious workforce shortage issues are predicted for most sectors of welfare care work, in aged care, nursing, and personal care for example. At present national governments in the more affluent societies are not scrupling to use immigrants from less affluent societies to plug the growing gaps in the supply of such workers. This can only postpone dealing with the real issue—how to create a sustainable economy of welfare work that is articulated with the public government of professional and para-professional education and training—and it is a solution bought at the expense of the integrity of poorer state-societies.

Perhaps even more importantly, and this will be true also of the better-paid categories of workers in a private service sector, there is nothing in the design of a private service market that offers containment for the emotional aspects of service work. As we have seen, if there is no support for the worker's capacity to contain the emotional aspects of service work, it is not likely that the worker will be able to sustain careful and individually-respectful as well as responsive care.

Facilitative government of publicly-oriented welfare services

Let me begin here with the issue of sustainability. A sustainable economy of welfare services must depend on the provision of funds, of course, but perhaps the most significant and intangible factor in enabling a sustainable economy of welfare services is the kind of good will that is associated with the desire to give or serve those who need what it is one has to offer. This is a desire not just associated with a professional service ethic. People who are not professionals but who are willing as relatives, neighbours, friends, and retirees with time on their hands, to lend a hand, maybe even to get a modicum of training to become someone who offers companionship to a person who needs it (a young person in care, someone with an intellectual disability who needs assistance in going to the movies, etc.), or offer an informal service are also to be considered here. Moreover, beyond the professionals and those who offer informal service, there are the individuals who need services themselves. Their good will is central to sustainable service delivery. An individual client who trusts that her individuality will be respected and recognized, that there is sufficient staffing continuity to ensure that there is continuity in responding to her needs, that the service will be reliable in the way she needs it to be, and that she is safe from abuse or domination in the service environment, is likely to cooperate with service provision out of good will. She is willing not just to be responsive in the way she needs to be but to be also creative in suggesting good-enough ways of responding to her needs, where she recognizes resource limits, and, generally, to work *with* the service providers so that it is a relationship both can value and enjoy.

Good will can be intelligently harnessed so that it informs an ethos of publicly-governed welfare service provision that inspires confidence and civic pride. If such an ethos is to be in play, government must honour those who provide good will in all these ways. It will champion the importance of a professional service ethic and provide a range of ways that make visible and honour all the different kinds of contribution people make to enhancing individual well-being. These would include a prominent valuing of self-advocacy programs for those who use welfare services especially but not only in the areas where stigma is still a problem for welfare service users (e.g. correctional services, mental health and children in care). Government must also consider how best to develop and support the institutions of professional education and training so as to cultivate a public ethic of professional service and autonomous professionalism. It must reintroduce the idea of substantial public subsidy for the costs of professional education and training in order to attract individuals to these career routes in exchange for a clear understanding that it will use its power to keep the costs of services down through a variety of mechanisms. For-profit providers of welfare services must understand that their business is subject to the regulation of government in the public interest.

For all of this to work government must open up a public sphere of informed discussion about welfare services where all the different stakeholders learn how to engage in regular conversation with each other, and, thus, learn how to appreciate the legitimacy of each others' different standpoint, and factor it into how they hold their own. Such a public sphere of sharing viewpoints and ideas about welfare services, and how they might continue to grow and develop, has to be independent of government's interest as both a policy making and funding agency in relation to welfare services. Somehow it has to be possible for those who represent these standpoints of government to come into public discussion with an honest ownership of their standpoint but in such a way that they can test and explore its possibilities as well as limits in relation to what it is the other stakeholders have to offer. In such discussion, the issues of resource scarcity can be publicly canvassed in such a way that the reality of this constraint can be both acknowledged and tested.

If the intangible factor of good will, shorthand for the remarkable ways in which people can open up possibilities of a situation if only they feel free and safe to do so, is to be in play, then ground-level service delivery has to function in an autonomous as well as accountable way. As Cooper and Lousada (2005, 41) argue, there has to be 'a clear point of demarcation between the arenas of practice and policy, in order that a genuine dialogue—or even contest—of ideas that a rooted in experience can take place at the boundary, or in the intermediate third area between the two'. Government's responsibility is to stabilize the policy, funding, and regulative environment of practice as well as to provide the structure for articulating issues and learning at ground-level into the policy process.

Finally, it is critical that government take responsibility for the public articulation of an ethic of personhood that is contextually appropriate. If welfare services can assume a wider governmental context that is oriented to securing the standing of all individuals who come under a particular governmental jurisdiction as persons, such ethical congruence invites welfare services to show what is possible to achieve in terms of facilitating the potential of individuals to achieve the status of a person who is capable of recognizing others as persons too.

At present, government has adopted a control rather than facilitative orientation to the world of welfare services. Instead of a stable government-provided environment of policy, funding and regulation, the opposite might be said to be the case. Consider this description from two US-based researchers on human service organizations which could be generalized to other contemporary jurisdictions:

> Since the 1980s, researchers have documented a human services sector rife with turmoil and crises. Many of the environmental challenges are the result of the continuing devolution, privatization and commercialization of social welfare policies and programs. These challenges include a decrease in resources accompanied by an increase in service demands, heightened competition among agencies, and greater emphasis on cost and performance accountability ... Many scholars and practitioners argue that social problems have become more complex and intractable, making them less resolvable particularly given the current preference for cost containment strategies. Demographic shifts also pose external concerns. The growth of populations of color, the elderly and people with disabilities present unique challenges to human service agencies such as a change in services offered or a retraining of staff (Hopkins and Hyde 2002, 2–3).

Questions of the delivery of welfare services are intimately linked to the larger question of whether at a societal level people are willing to engage in the kind of learning that promotes a sustainable, public and ethical response to the management of complexity and uncertainty. The fate of welfare services might be said to concern the sustainability of the internal world of human society, a fate surely profoundly connected to the sustainability of human society's external 'natural' world.

Part II
The Case Studies

8
Public Bureaucracy and 'Customer Service': The Case of Centrelink 1996–2004

Anna Yeatman

It is often assumed that public bureaucracy is inherently antagonistic to the individualization of the delivery of welfare services. In this chapter I make not only the argument that such an assumption is incorrect and betrays an animus towards public bureaucracy (for discussion see Du Gay 2000, Introduction) but I offer a case study of how a public bureaucracy was remodelled in terms of the contemporary ethos of customer service, understood as a public rather than a private ethos.

The creation of Centrelink as a statutory 'service delivery' agency

In 1996 the newly elected conservative Australian government led by Prime Minister John Howard took as one of its first initiatives the establishment of a one-stop shop for the provision of government services. While the largest component of these services was to be 'the administration of entitlements under social security legislation', the new agency was to 'deliver services for a number of portfolios and integrate these into a common point of customer contact': 'it will provide an administrative framework for integrating access to Commonwealth services by consolidating services so that, where possible, people can get the help they need in one place (Second Reading, Commonwealth Services Delivery Agency Bill 1996)'. Here is Minister Ruddock's provision of the rationale for the new agency in the Second Reading of the Bill:

> The government's objectives in creating the agency are to provide a much better standard of service delivery to the community and to

individuals; and to increase service delivery efficiency and effectiveness. The government wishes to shift the focus and direction of customer service from the mechanics of transaction and process to one which is centred on individuals and their needs. The scope of the agency's activities will cover services to the retired, families, the unemployed, carers and widows, the short-term incapacitated and people with disabilities. It will be the public presence for some of the most sensitive social responsibilities of government.

The new agency was called Centrelink, and its founding Chief Executive Officer was Sue Vardon whom we meet again in Chapter 13 (in her earlier capacity as CEO of South Australian Corrections). Besides the service delivery rationale for its existence, the new agency was also to reduce duplication and inefficiencies in previous arrangements in a context where the Government had decided also to contract out job-placement services to a network of private providers (Rowlands 1999, 226). The administrative rationalization aspect of the new arrangement addressed 'a long-standing issue', namely, 'the existence of separate networks of regional offices of the Department of Education, Employment, Training and Youth Affairs (DEETYA) and DSS' (Halligan 2006, 88). Now these two networks were collapsed and integrated into the new agency.

Established as a statutory agency with its own board, Centrelink was placed in a contractual, purchaser-provider relationship to its client government departments. John Halligan (2006, 88) explains this rather ambiguous situation of Centrelink in relation to the line management authority of a government department as follows:

> The original concept ... was of an agency that would ... have two major clients, but serve others. Centrelink is located within the core public service and [prior to 2004] within the Family and Community Services [FaCS] portfolio, but it is an entity separate from the FaCS department, with its own legislation, accounting, and reporting requirements.

Right from the start the new CEO ran hard with the mandate for the new organization as one focused on service delivery: customer service. In particular, she emphasized the importance of shifting the model of service delivery from a bureaucratic 'stovepipe' model, where the program was conceived and shaped in terms of its relationship to the specific policy it was designed to implement, to one that was adapted to the needs of citizens. Here is Sue Vardon's explanation in 1999 of the difference between these two models:

> Prior to the creation of Centrelink government services were not integrated. Entitlements were delivered through several largely independent government agencies. Customers were slotted into the appropriate income support streams. Staffing, office workflow practices and the systems that staff used in their day to day work were configured on program or payment lines.
>
> With the creation of Centrelink we undertook a range of customer research. This involved nearly 9000 customers in some specific feedback workshops with Centrelink staff. It continues. Having listened to our customers we realised that this model did not respond to individuals or the complexities of their life circumstances. Customers also told us they didn't care which department was responsible and they didn't necessarily care what the products were called. They just want to be able to tell us their circumstances and to be offered the best package of products and services to which they are entitled that will meet their individual needs (Vardon 1999b, 2–3).

For as long as she remained CEO (1997–2004), Sue Vardon did all she could to realize the brief outlined in the Second Reading for the Bill establishing the new agency. The initiative deserves the encomium given it by Carmen Zanetti (1998) when she was National Manager, Strategic Services, Centrelink, Australia:

> It is a unique model of public administration in human services in the world. The Centrelink approach shifts the focus and direction of customer service from transactions and processes framed by the boundaries of Commonwealth departments and agencies, to one that is centred on individuals and their needs.

In championing customer service, Centrelink was positioned in a tricky relationship to the two principal policy departments engaged in purchasing services from Centrelink: FaCS and the successor to DEETYA, DEWR (Department of Employment and Workplace Relations). Centrelink was not just implementing the policy of these departments but had a legislative mandate to engage in an orientation of customer service to the members of the public. Centrelink considered it had responsibility for advising its client departments on how their policy impacted on its customers, and thus began to adopt a policy advising role, while these client departments understood their role to be that of policy, Centrelink's role that of 'delivery' (for discussion of this tension see Halligan 2006). Centrelink under Vardon's leadership championed the idea of a strategic partnership between it and its principal government departments. In fact, Centrelink and FaCS evolved a partnership approach, but this did not obviate the ambiguity in the relationship nor the central agency (Department of Finance) view that the purchaser/provider model based in agency theory is the one that should prevail, where the relationship between FaCS and Centrelink was seen as insufficiently at arm's length (Halligan 2006, 94).

There was also a strong and unresolvable tension between an ethos of customer service, on the one hand, and a conservative government's readiness to use populist rhetoric of dole-cheats and welfare-bludgers as well as to tighten the compliance requirements for the individual recipient of income support, using desktop computer applications to enforce not just accuracy in payment but rule-following procedure on administrative staff, and putting considerable effort into identifying and punishing 'welfare cheats'.[1] It is possible to adopt a facilitation of compliance approach, one that was recommended in 1997 by Jocelyn Pech, a policy analyst at that time in the Department of Social Security, who proposed with regard to 'the activity test' for unemployed people on income support:

> ... the prevailing view is that it is a tool of compliance and control. However, there is an alternative more positive view—that its primary purpose is to help unemployed people back to work by providing a guide to activities seen as useful for achieving this goal. This view emphasises the test's helping role rather than its role to prescribe behaviour (Pech 1997, 3).

The purchasing department responsible for employment services, Department of Employment and Workplace Relations (DEWR), consistently took more of a control than a facilitation of compliance approach to the public management of people on unemployment benefits and could see only one model of 'participation': participation in the labour market economy. This Department practiced a form of 'splitting' (in the psychoanalytic sense of the word) in using in-house language that distinguished between 'the cuddlies' (older people who are seen as legitimate long-term income support beneficiaries) and 'the non-cuddlies' (people deemed employable and therefore not seen as legitimate income support beneficiaries).[2] On the other hand, the department responsible for purchasing most of the income support services from Centrelink, Family and Community Services (FaCS), was friendly to a customer focus orientation and to a more encompassing idea of participation, but at the same time, *vis-à-vis* Centrelink, was protective of its policy turf.

There was a third tension between the business model proposed for the new service delivery agency which was expressed in giving it a governing board that included four members from the private sector along with the two departmental secretaries and Centrelink's CEO, and direct ownership of the agency by government. The board was justifiably interested in entrepreneurship on behalf of the new agency, and it had a direct relationship to the minister for the Centrelink portfolio, but this could readily cut across established departmental lines of bureaucratic responsibility and accountability. In part, this third tension related to the fourth: that between government's interest as an owner and its interest as a funder of services (discussed by Rowlands 1999, 228). As a funder or purchaser of services, government's interest is in getting the best value for money, which may cut across the cost of long-term investment in public infrastructure for income support services. Rowlands explains:

> One of the most significant assets in the custody of Centrelink is the computer system it uses to deliver services. If we contemplate that asset from the perspective of the owner, we would like to see it maintained at a very high level of integrity, completeness and reliability. When a client department wants to make a change to a program or introduce a new one, they are likely to press for the least costly option consistent with reasonable reliability. However, the owner is likely to want changes to the technical systems to be made in a way that best satisfies Centrelink's proper role and future capability as a one-stop shop. That is, they will tend to want wherever possible, the more comprehensive approach, the one that best positions Centrelink for its long-term function. This would especially be the case in a contestable environment where Centrelink would be expected to make financial returns to its owner on the owner's investment. The trouble is, this is likely to be a more expensive option than the purchaser would choose. Under pressure to minimise the cost of current budget options, the purchaser may see little short-run incentive to invest in the

capacity of the provider to produce future output. So how do we balance government-as-owner with government-as-purchaser? (Rowlands 1999, 228–229).

Sue Vardon resigned as CEO in 2004.[3] This was the year that the Howard Government reconsidered the standing of Centrelink as an agency with its own governing board. It abolished the board, and placed Centrelink as a statutory agency within an umbrella 'Human Services' government department responsible as the 'core department' for managing Centrelink along with the Child Support Agency, the Health Insurance Commission, Australian Hearing, Commonwealth Rehabilitation Services Australia, and Health Services Australia. By this time the Government had intensified its 'welfare to work' demands now extended to sole parent and disability income support beneficiaries whereas when Centrelink was set up there was more acceptance in government policy that sole parents were engaged in a major social contribution, parenting, at least until their last child was of school age, and that many people on disability support pensions were not fit for regular and sustained employment. The first annual report of the new CEO of Centrelink under the new arrangement, Jeff Whalan, not only indicates that the Welfare to Work program is firmly under the control of DEWR, thus representing a shift in the balance of power from FaCS to DEWR as client agencies, but that the major challenge of Centrelink for 2005–2006 'will be to successfully introduce the Welfare to Work initiatives and to assist as many people as possible to access work (*Centrelink* 2005, Chapter One)'.

In November 2007, the Howard Government lost power and was replaced by the Rudd Labor Government. At the time of writing this chapter, it is too soon to say how the policy context for Centrelink may be reshaped by the new government, but one thing seems already clear, a shift away from giving policy priority to the pursuit of 'welfare cheats', a pursuit that seems to have become obsessive once DEWR became responsible for the expanded pool of people now subject to the regime of 'welfare to work' (see Jopson and Horin 2007).

The focus of this chapter is on the conception of customer service developed by Centrelink under the leadership of Sue Vardon between its establishment and 2003 when my fieldwork ended. More attention will be given to the conception than to its implementation because at the time of completion of fieldwork it is fair to say that the conception while complete was still in the early stages of being implemented on an organization-wide basis. Just to give some sense of the scale of

Centrelink as reported by its CEO in 2003 (Vardon 2003), it administered 9.3 million entitlements to 6.4 million customers; its transactions included 28.9 million webpage views by people going into its website, 6.5 million appointments and 22.5 million calls to 28 call centres; its budget was AUD 53 billion; it produced over 140 products and services; and it was engaging in public business on behalf of 25 client (government) departments or agencies.

My fieldwork took the form of interviews with Sue Vardon (who read this chapter in draft, offered no revisions of the account I offer of this history, and also consented to the use of her name)[4] and six other senior players in the formation and development of Centrelink from its inception, interviews with senior officials in FaCS, the collection of documents (including Sue Vardon's speeches), a presentation to the Centrelink Guiding Coalition, and participation in a Centrelink workshop on the introduction of 'personal advisers'.

Bureaucracy and customer service

The reorientation of public bureaucracy within an ethos of customer service should be seen as a reform movement within public administration. Bureaucracy continues to be the only appropriate ethical administrative structure of the state (for elaboration of this argument see Du Gay 2000 and 2005). Contrary to those who argue for the privatization of erstwhile public services so that they are transferred from state ownership to a market-based model of service provision, the inherent ethos of public bureaucracy lends itself to this kind of reform. The case for reform is well put by Michael Keating (2001, 99), former head of the Australian Public Service and of various senior Departments including Prime Minister and Cabinet under the Hawke, Keating and Howard governments:

> The main thrust of reforms has been to shift from an hierarchical system of decision-making, based on precedence and compliance with rules. This system may have worked well enough a century or more ago when government's interaction with citizens was principally directed to ensuring their equal treatment before the law. It was, however, bound to change as society became more diverse and increasingly rejected the notion that 'one size fits all'. Governments accordingly came under pressure to be more responsive to changing citizen demands and expectations. Moreover, the original justification for many of the old rules had long been lost sight of and they

were largely being followed for their own sake. Public servants engaged in service delivery were essentially process driven and found it difficult to say what it was that they were actually trying to achieve.

Citizens have become more rather than less dependent on state-provided services, a trajectory that accompanies the twentieth century expansion of public responsibility for welfare services broadly understood (see Chapter 1 for this conception of welfare) and for public infrastructure. It is not just citizens it is all people who come under the jurisdiction of a particular state who are dependent on state provision of services in one way or another, even allowing for how difference between the statuses of citizen, permanent resident, temporary resident and illegal alien affect eligibility for different kinds of public service. In interview, Sue Vardon spoke of Jocelyn Newman, the government minister whose portfolio made her responsible for the establishment of Centrelink, as having 'a huge passion for the citizen'. Here is the relevant part of the interview transcript referring to the political will of both Prime Minister Howard and Minister Newman in getting Centrelink created:

Jocelyn Newman ... was very connected to her community of Tasmania [the smallest state in Australia]. And old ladies [old age pensioners] would come up to her and say 'that letter that they sent to me that says ... if I don't tell you my change of address ... there'll be a fine of two thousand dollars if I don't do it or six months in gaol. My husband fought in the war, I've built Australia, I've had six kids, why would you send me to gaol?' And of course ... she would get cross ... and she kept hearing these stories about poor service ... I don't believe in visions, she said, Sue, I'm not into that vision stuff. She had a strong social policy view but ... beneath [that] a vision for the improvement of service delivery ... this agency that she created—she referred to it as 'her agency'— ... 'was going to be respectful and ... would treat the person as a citizen', ... that was very much part of her. ... I use the word 'citizen' because we have such comprehensive cover, but a million of our customers aren't citizens so it's a bit of a problem, so I go in and out of different languages.

Minister Newman, thus, placed herself in the vanguard of those who have sought to shift a traditionalist public bureaucracy operating in terms of precedent and customary practice into a more reflexive and post-paternalistic mode of operating in relation to citizens. Her emphasis is congruent with the relevant section of 'Australian Public Service Values' in the new 1999 Australian Public Service Act: 'the APS delivers services fairly, effectively, impartially and courteously to the Australian public and is sensitive to the diversity of the Australian public'. As we shall see this approach is one that ensures that the formal entitlement of people to public income support and related services, instead of being hidden away in arcane bureaucratic rules that are interpreted by public servants, is to become publicly available and readily accessible information. This is in line with the fundamental principles of publicly accountable, transparent and impartial government enunciated by John Locke in the seventeenth century: 'For all the power the Government has, being only for the good of the Society, as it ought not to be Arbitrary and at Pleasure, so it ought to be exercised by established and promulgated Laws: that both the People may know their Duty, and be safe and secure within the limits of the Law, and the Rulers too kept within their due bounds, and not be tempted by the Power they have in their hands, to imploy it to such purposes, and by such measures, as they would not have known, and own not willingly (Locke 1970, 360, emphasis in original).'

The new emphases in the contemporary conception of public service values are on citizen diversity and the value of service itself. These emphases do not challenge the ethos of public bureaucracy so much as remake it to fit the contemporary historical context. Paul Du Gay (2005) argues for the continuing relevance of Max Weber's conception of bureaucracy as a 'non-sectarian comportment of the person', one that is able to administer affairs of state in a neutral, impartial and procedurally-correct way. As Paul Hoggett, building on Du Gay's (2000) argument, suggests, the bureaucratic virtues of impartiality and impersonality is an inherently 'individualizing' orientation to those who as citizen/ non-citizen-subjects come within the ambit of public bureaucratic - administration:

> [Du Gay] argues that the value attached to impersonality by Weber must be understood as itself being an expression of democratic equalization and therefore a more ethically advanced form of authority than that based on personal considerations ('grace and favour', nepotism, cronyism, etc.) which characterized

organizational life in public and private spheres before the quicken-
ing of modernization in the early twentieth century. In other words,
the impartiality of the bureaucrat entails 'a trained capacity to
treat people as "individual" cases, that is, apart from status and
ascription' (Hoggett 2005b, 173).

It is this impartiality of the public bureaucrat that enables people
to be treated as individuals who are each entitled to being regarded
as a person or subject of right, to use the language I used in Chapter 3.
At the same time, government in its role as the public authority (the
other term for this is 'the state') legitimately requires those subject
to its jurisdiction to accept its authority and to provide the taxation
basis of its revenue. For this reason, government provision of service is
never separable from particular requirements of citizen compliance
with law and administrative procedure. Thus if in contemporary
rhetoric for public service we find the idea of serving the customer,
it is important to situate the term 'customer' within a public rather
than private ethical setting.

Centrelink as a customer service organization

If one of the drivers of the creation of Centrelink was political
will, another was a push for administrative efficiency by merging
what had been two distinct bureaucratic service delivery networks
(income support and some job seeker services provided by the Department of Social Security and the Commonwealth Employment Service
respectively), thus achieving cost savings. In addition to being positioned as a monopoly provider of such services, Centrelink could
be selected as a service portal by other government departments,
or it could tender for their business.[5] In some cases, it could enter
partnership with other government services to become a comprehensive one-stop shop. As a service portal, for example, Centrelink
has been responsible for drought assistance to farmers, and after
the Bali bombings, it provided a 24-hour hotline for survivors and
their families; and, as an example of inter-governmental partnership, Centrelink entered a partnership with Service Tasmania, the
Tasmanian Government's shopfront in ten rural and regional
locations: 'Customers in seven of these sites can access Commonwealth, State and local government services from the one Service Tasmania shop (*Centrelink Annual Review 2000–2001*, no
pagination)'.

Centrelink was expected to serve both its 'client' Departments and its individual 'customers'. At first there was some ambiguity concerning the Government's intention regarding its continuing ownership of Centrelink, there being some suggestion it might contract out this set of service delivery functions, and thus in its 1998–1999 *Annual Report*, Centrelink indicates that its first 'business outcome' is to 'be first choice of Government for the provision of government services (Centrelink 1998–1999, 6).'[6] Thus in order to demonstrate it should continue to receive funding from the purchasing government departments, Centrelink has to establish that it was both effective and efficient as a service delivery agency. Zanetti (1998, 6) comments: 'The fact that Centrelink's funds come through contracts and not directly from government brings a strong discipline on performance management and business partnership'.

In interview, Sue Vardon said that she was clear from the outset that the first task was to create a vision for the new organization. In this she was influenced by John Kotter's conception of leading change in business firms; in interview, she said that she had been familiar with this approach since her work in South Australian Corrections (see Chapter 13). Kotter (1995) recommends eight steps for transforming an organization: establishing a sense of urgency; forming a powerful guiding coalition; creating a vision; communicating the vision; empowering others to act on the vision; planning for and creating short-term wins; consolidating improvements and producing still more change; and institutionalizing new approaches. Vardon was clear there needed to be a common vision expressed in common language. From the outset Centrelink committed to the methodology of value creation workshops in order to seek direct customer feedback. Value creation workshops are a form of 'customer-driven research' described by the two developers of this approach in Australia as follows:

> Customer-driven research is a means of establishing customer values whilst avoiding the imposition of the researcher's perceptual set upon the customer's thinking. It questions the assumption that all customers want 'improved quality'—as defined by the designers of products and services—because, not all customers perceive value in 'so-called' quality improvements. The replacement assumption is that customers know what they value and can describe the ideal service; and, furthermore, that customers can and should become

partners in the improvement process (Bennington and Cummane 1997, 89).

A value-creation workshop brings together both agency customers and service staff. It is described in the Centrelink handout on 'Value Creation in Centrelink: an introduction' as follows:

> Value Creation Workshops allow customers to provide direct feedback about the services they receive, creating an opportunity for service providers to:
>
> • Hear first-hand what their customers think about the service they are providing;
> • Put themselves in their customers' shoes (by trying to anticipate what it is that the customer values, or finds irritating, about doing business with Centrelink, and how the customers rate the current service); and
> • Use the feedback to plan for local service improvement.

By the end of July 1998 the agency, established in 1997, had involved 6,920 customers and 9,885 staff in 525 workshops (Zanetti 1998, 8). The use of value creation workshops to develop the language of customer service and the culture of listening to the customer within Centrelink was clearly central to Vardon's strategy for building the new service organization. Such data was triangulated with surveys of customer satisfaction which included a biannual national telephone survey and a survey of general community awareness and views of Centrelink (Vardon 1999b, 7).

The language of 'customer'

The language of 'customer' for service recipients was adopted from the outset. When asked in interview why she had used this term rather than say 'consumer', Vardon responded:

> AY: Why customer rather than consumer?
> SV: For me the word consumer has an eating connotation [laughs] … No, why customer was because Social Security had used it and … I actually didn't care. I just knew there was going to be a debate and my … public statement is, look, I don't actually care about the language, please, don't argue about the language, so long as my people

call people by their names—Mr Smith, or you know, hello George—that's much more important. … we have of course client departments who are our customers, consider themselves to be the dominant customer, and, [then], the citizen. So instead of calling it customer and citizen, we said client and customer. But they are both equally important … in the end it's jargon … it's language … I can't ever keep everybody happy, so we made a choice. But I thought, I'll use a word that thousands of people are used to … The CES people of course had clients and hated to come over to customers. So I said, you want to keep on calling them clients, you just do that, I don't care. So … to this day you can tell the difference between a CES person and a DSS person by the language they use inside [the organization].

The value creation workshops established early and consistently feedback from Centrelink customers that Vardon could use to validate new points of leadership for the organization. Such feedback became known as 'customer values':

Customers have consistently told us that these are the top six things they would value from a 'best in the world service'

- Friendly, helpful and caring staff.
- Prompt and efficient service—and to tell my story only once.
- An integrated service which gets positive outcomes.
- Easy access, choice of access.
- Skilled and knowledgeable staff.
- A welcoming and comfortable office environment.

From the outset of the new organization, Vardon emphasized the language of customer: 'we introduced the "Customer" everywhere—customer services officers instead of counter assessors; customer service centres instead of regional offices; customer segment teams instead of policy or program branches (Vardon 1999b, 10)'. The customer service centres were physically transformed—'down came the high counters and back offices to be replaced by modern open offices where all staff have a public contact desk'; 'the numbered ticketing system for customer interviews was replaced by the opportunity to make a pre-booked interview'; all staff were asked to wear their name badge in order to establish 'a more personalised approach, accountability and [to] instil … confidence that the person wearing the organization's logo bearing their name is a professional service officer (Vardon 1999b, 10)'.

A new service delivery model

The organization also developed a new service delivery model so that at the point of contact between citizen-customer and the agency, the 'service offer' was conceived in terms of what made sense to customers rather than what made sense to policy makers and program managers. In Cohen's (2002) terms, this is to adopt an approach that groups service units and staff by 'market' rather than 'function'. Functional structures are organized in terms of specialized areas and thus they tend to have a 'silo' effect where it is difficult to produce seamless flow or coordination across areas (Cohen 2002, 27). A market grouping approach, on the other hand, follows from the needs of those whom the organization serves. This became the basis of the 'life events' approach to grouping Centrelink's products and services that was introduced in 1998; it was overlaid on a customer segment approach, a functional structure, where staff were grouped in terms of programs—youth and students, families and children, people of workforce age, retirees, and people with disabilities and their carers (Ross 2003, 22). With the 'life events' approach, staff were expected to be able to think across programs in response to a customer's needs. As Vardon (1999b) puts it: 'this approach ... has us tipping the bureaucracy upside down to present an approach to service delivery from the customer's point of view'. In interview, she said that she found the life events approach through experience both of a hospital in Britain and Harrods:

> ... the hospital in Britain ... did something fabulous. ... if you have arthritis, you can go and have a touch screen and everything about arthritis was available to you: where the doctors were, what was a symptom, what food you should be eating ... and they would package it all up about arthritis. And I thought ... that's interesting. And then Harrods ... decided they were going to put all their packaging around events. So ... if you wanted to ... get something for a person's twenty-first birthday party, you could see a range of gifts and also buy your shoes and the dress for the night ... and the tie for your partner and whatever ... They packaged the event of the twenty-first birthday party. So I met a woman from England and I said I think there's a life event concept here ... and we started to build it ...

The 'life events' are classified into 12 possibilities in response to the question 'How can Centrelink help you?' which include such things as 'planning your retirement?', 'seeking or changing education?', 'in a crisis situation?', and 'sick or disabled?' They provide a framework for Centrelink staff in designing a service offer that is tailored to the particular customer's situation which may not fit into any one of the customer segments. Sheila Ross (2003, 22) explains: 'Overlaid in the [customer segment] construct is the "life events" model where we acknowledge that a customer's circumstances do not fit neatly into one or other of these segments (for example, people of any age may ask for our assistance about housing or relationship problems) and seek to connect them with the range of payments and services that apply in their situation.'

Also Centrelink gave considerable attention to using new information and communication technologies to create both easy access and also choice of point of access ('channel') for customers. It developed call centres that linked into customer service centres thus enabling call centre staff to transfer a customer call to someone in a customer service centre. Each customer had a single, integrated, computer-based file. The old paper-based manuals outlining the fine print of eligibility for program access and other policy requirements that were cumbersome and arcane by any standards were replaced by a computer based system—an e-reference suite—that makes it easy for the customer service officer to input data on their desktop computer about an individual customer and get an immediate response concerning eligibility. The agency's public website was redesigned for easy access to information about services as framed by the life events approach, eligibility, and other relevant aspects of Centrelink operations. All of this was done in the name of both customer service and 'transparency'. In interview, Sue Vardon commented (this being in 2003):

> The first thing we'll do is send our e-reference suite out to thousands of community organizations so they can print it off for a customer. And eventually you'll be able to get it off the website ... Transparency is a fundamental belief around here. We don't like secrets ... in fact I'm allergic to secrets. I've kept the budget stuff quietly in my mind [there was to be a major new budget announcement that would extend Centrelink's IT capabilities in the time following the interview], that's appropriate, but it's about the only kind of secret that I'll hold.

The replacement of paper manuals by the e-reference suite was the material basis for new expectations of how staff handled eligibility determination. In interview Sue Vardon said of the old Social Security culture that staff were not problem solvers:

> Social Security people were ... linear thinkers: are you eligible or ... not? They were not given the latitude to solve a problem, and in fact there was ... a legal [requirement of them] which was do not say 'you might be eligible for that', if they haven't asked for it because you might ... have forgotten to say 'and that and that and that', and they could sue you for failing a duty of care. So you only dealt with the request that came directly from the customer, it was [the customer's] responsibility to find other options. I said this is the most bizarre concept I've every heard in my life. It was the lifeblood of Social Security's thinking.

Personalized service

'Personalized' service is not the same as 'customized' or 'tailored' service. In the latter case, the service is designed so that it can be adapted to the particular profile of an individual customer. In the former case, the customer is led to believe that s/he will get 'personal' service from a particular service worker who continues to be 'his' or 'her' worker. In the interest of attempting to meet this goal, and also to enable customers to tell their story only once, Centrelink introduced a 'one main contact' model as Sue Vardon was calling it in 2003, it being earlier called a 'one-to-one' approach. The 1998–1999 *Annual Report* (Centrelink 1999, 39) stated this initiative 'involves every customer having one main Customer Service officer who manages all the business that a customer cannot do over the phone'. Sue Vardon (2000, 11) explains it thus:

> One-to-one service means that when people come to us they are allocated an individual Centrelink officer who can be their main point of contact with Centrelink. Our staff are each allocated a group of existing customers. New customers are progressively added to their portfolio. Staff accept responsibility for all ongoing business relating to their own customers ... Simple customer enquiries continue to be handled by Call Centre or reception staff.

The intention was to roll out this approach to service across all teams by the end of 1999; it presupposed that all work backlogs had been dealt with first. According to data collected by Cosmo Howard for three

Centrelink customer service centres in 2000–2001 in Canberra, Newcastle, and inner-city Melbourne respectively, this initiative met with difficulties owing mostly to high caseloads but also to customer 'no-shows' (Howard 2006, 149–150). Howard interestingly comments further that some of the customers he interviewed were not interested in the one-to-one service approach:

> One suggested that he tried to avoid appointments by finding a job and going off payments whenever he was called in for a meeting with Centrelink. Another asked to see the next available person, because he was more concerned about being seen quickly than seeing the same officer. ... the universalisation of the identity of the job seeker as a demanding individual requiring intensive personalised service does not always correspond with the orientations of recipients. Some beneficiaries did not regard themselves as unique individuals with particular problems needing holistic support and in-depth intervention (Howard 2006, 150).

I did not clarify where Sue Vardon thought this approach had got to in interview with her in 2003, but it seems clear that by then the 'triage' approach of the organization which classified customers into three groups had already overtaken the one-to-one approach to all customers. The triage approach is expressed as 'three ways that customers want to be serviced':

- **'Just do it'**—transactional response, often able to be completed through technological means.
- **'Help me'**—need to 'fix a problem', usually requiring combination of people and technology.
- **'Relate to me'**—requiring 'person focused solution' based on good understanding of circumstances and need at the time (Vardon 2003).

Internal organizational design and development for customer service

Sue Vardon was clear that the employees of Centrelink could not be expected to respect and listen to customers if they were not themselves respected and listened to within the organization. She was aware also of the importance of training staff; the organization developed a nationally accredited training program. She adopted the maxim, 'recruit for attitudes, train for skills' (Vardon 2000, 6). In order to create an organization with an open, transparent culture of listening and learning she did a number of things, of which I will select three: the flattening of the organization and the adoption of a team-based approach to organizational development; the creation of the Guiding Coalition (this being another of John Kotter's recommendations), and the creation of 'shared behaviours' as the basis of the culture of interaction between Centrelink staff. All of these changes occurred early in the new agency's life; they were clearly seen by Vardon as the foundations of building a new organization.

Recalling that Centrelink represented a merger between two preexisting bureaucracies, Vardon not only had to create a single, integrated organization but, as she saw it, to shift 'a traditional management' approach to one of shared leadership:

> On joining Centrelink I found a structure of fiefdoms and silos with communication going up and down the silos not across. Many of my senior people had not been directly involved in senior decision making and people at all levels were fearful—fearful of making mistakes—which meant we were not capturing their potential … People needed to understand the broader organization they worked in and the impact of their work on it. They needed to break free of the constraining silos, which are part and parcel of traditional bureaucracy, and, very importantly, they needed to have ownership of their work (Vardon 2000, 3).

Accordingly, she 'flattened the Senior Executive Service (SES) structure, doing away with divisions and branches and created teams' where a SES officer 'leads each team' (Vardon 2000, 3). 'There is no pecking order to these teams and their leaders'—'We created a collegiate group of peers' (Vardon 2000, 3). Each team leader was a co-eval member of the collegiate group which was called the Guiding Coalition. In interview, Vardon agreed that the Guiding Coalition could be described as 'the mind' of the organization. She said that she needed to shift the organization out of a 'command/control environment' and, instead of a hierarchy of vertically integrated organizational segments, ensure that there was horizontal communication across the different areas of the organization: the IT people, the field people, the operations people, the Canberra-based people, the regional-centre people, and so on. The Guiding Coalition (GC) began from the outset as an executive-level team-based approach to leading the organization. Vardon represented the GC as Centrelink's 'internal Corporate Board': 'there are 60 or so members who meet every six weeks and, whenever possible, away from Canberra (our national capital and central administration for most major government agencies'), thus giving the GC 'the opportunity to visit the local customer service centres to learn from the people who are so important to the survival of our organisation—the staff who serve our customers' (Vardon 2003, 3). Not only would it have been impossible to develop the IT possibilities of Centrelink without horizontal integration of this kind, Vardon knew that a customer service organization could not be developed 'by direction' (interview data). By 2003 (Vardon 2003, 3), she argued the GC 'has become a very strong body'. My own impression when I gave a presentation to the GC in May that same year was that it was an open dialogical environment that invited a learning or enquiry mode, and where it seemed that all were confident in offering their views or questions, and not looking to the CEO's approval. Vardon (2003, 3) commented further:

> One of my colleagues commented that through the Guiding Coalition for the first time in her career she now knows what is going on. No decisions behind closed doors. She feels empowered because she has the information and has the opportunity to have her say.

'Shared behaviours' was a set of expectations for how Centrelink staff interacted with each other (these being the 'internal' customers) and with their external customers. The behaviours were (from Vardon 2003, 10):

- Listening—listen to customers and the community
- Problem solving—solve problems and develop opportunities
- Exploring—explore and put in place innovative and cost effective ways to provide the right outcome
- Behaving—behave with integrity and in an ethical manner
- Respecting—display mutual respect for our customers and each other

In interview, Sue Vardon said the 'shared behaviours' were posted everywhere: 'You bump into them everywhere in a Centrelink [office]' (interview data). She said further that they 'were established early and they've been very important, in fact somebody recently said, well, isn't it time to review them and there was a universal resistance to touching them'.

On being asked whether in the Guiding Coalition there are protocols for listening, Vardon referred to the shared behaviours:

> ... people don't interrupt each other, people will say, hang on, that's not a shared behaviour, if they over-talk each other. ... sometimes I think, oh my god, what have I created? (interview data).

Conclusion

The story of Centrelink 1997 until the departure of its first CEO Sue Vardon in 2004 is a fascinating combination of populist as well as citizenship-oriented politics, administrative rationalization, and the personal effectiveness of a visionary public servant in building a team-based approach to a customer service organization. Vardon followed John Kotter's lessons for building an effective organization that is able to respond creatively to a challenging environment. Kotter (1995, 66) makes it clear that 'until changes sink deeply into a company's culture, a process that can take five to ten years, new approaches are fragile and subject to regression'. With Vardon's leaving, prompted as it was by the Howard Government's pulling Centrelink back into a regular hier-archical relationship to a home government Department, it seems unlikely that the vision Vardon pursued so deliberately and congru-ently had time to bed down. As already said, in 2004 the Howard Government began to ratchet up an emphasis on a 'welfare-to-work' approach to the provision of income support to a widening group of people deemed employable and, as it did this, there would be an inevitable tension between asking of Centrelink front counter staff that they engage in a customer service ethos while simultaneously enforc-ing the new 'participation' requirements. It seems clear from newspa-per reportage that there has been post-Vardon a shift in Centrelink's *modus operandi* from a facilitation of compliance approach to one of control. Stephanie Peatling in a *Sydney Morning Herald* article (January 15 2008) cites a letter to the Ombudsman from the CEO of Centrelink, Jeff Whalan, which revealed that in the 2006–2007 financial year, 525,654 'participation failures' were submitted to Centrelink for inves-tigation by Job Network agencies (responsible for the provision of job placement services).

If Vardon's approach was difficult to accommodate within a harsher policy regime for people receiving income support who were deemed employable, it was also out of sync with the hierarchical administra-tive culture of Canberra-based government Departments. Vardon saw promise in the new administrative arrangement by which Centrelink as the service delivery agency was differentiated from the policy agencies that purchased Centrelink's services. However, from interview data and other sources (Halligan 2006; Zanetti 1998) it is clear that Vardon's emphasis was on a 'differentiation' of roles as well as a strategic partnership between Centrelink and its 'client' departments, rather than on the control and command relationship that is assumed by agency theory. In agency theory, in purchasing 'the agent's' services, 'the principal' has the right to command the agent, and the entire relationship is set up in order to permit the principal as much effective control over the agent as possible (for agency theory, see Boston *et al*. 18–21; Althaus 1997; Perrow 1986). Vardon rejected the agency theory approach to the relationship between purchasing policy department and the service delivery agency (interview data). She thought what happened on the ground in terms of service delivery should inform the evolution and revision of policy. It is likely that she would be sympathetic to Paul Hoggett's (2005, 176) view that 'the dogma separating policy from [its] execution must be challenged', and that 'in reality, policy issues exist at all levels, even the management of a [public-local government owned] swimming pool poses complex policy questions—are there reserved sessions for older users or for Asian women, how much time should be allocated to club use as opposed to general use, etc.?' Elsewhere I have contrasted an *executive model* of the policy process, that positions the service delivery arm of government in a strictly instrumental relationship of implementation of policy as determined by the executive levels of government with a *co-production model* of the policy process, where the service delivery arm is invited into a shared process of problem-setting and problem-solving with those responsible for establishing policy direction for a program (Yeatman 1998a). Halligan's (2006, 93) comments are suggestive of how much Vardon's approach incited resistance from the two main purchasing departments, FaCS and DEWR:

> The main purchasing departments, FaCS and Employment and Workplace Relations, accepted a role for Centrelink in providing advice on the delivery aspects of specific policy proposals. That role was regarded as secondary ... However, opposition to leading on policy agenda was strong. Centrelink should be consulted and should argue very forcibly in terms of the implementation of the policy agenda. And that may even mean that the policy agenda gets

... amended ... But I don't think they 'should be taking the initiative in terms of driving policy' (Senior departmental official).

In light of this, it may come as no surprise that in the *2004–2005 Annual Report* of DEWR, there is a (surely deliberate) reversal of Centrelink language. In the section called 'Departmental Values' and in dot point form, we find: 'our Ministers are our primary customers', while jobseekers, Indigenous communities and employers' employees are 'our primary clients'.

Notes

1   In the Short Form overview of its *Annual Review 2002–2003*, Centrelink in a section titled 'Protecting the integrity of outlays', refers to its role as 'one of ensuring that the approximately $55 billion we pay out to our customers is paid correctly', and goes on to say that its compliance activities 'are specifically aimed at the prevention, detection and deterrence of incorrect payments and fraud to ensure customers are receiving their correct entitlements'. These activities include: identity checks, data-matching with information held by Centrelink or obtained from other agencies; tip-offs provided by the public; inter-agency compliance activities; selecting customers for review on the basis of risk or as part of random sample surveys'.
2   This information was given to the research team for this project by someone in Centrelink in 2006.
3   The Centrelink media release for her resignation is dated 10 November 2004.
4   In her email to me indicating her responses to the draft chapter, she added 'I am always conscious that it wasn't just me—lots of other people shaped the organization'.
5   In a handout of PowerPoint slides prepared for a talk in Canada (Vardon 2003), one slide outlines the three ways Centrelink gets its business: (1) as preferred provider—from its original charter; (2) as convenient supplier—as in the case of drought and the Bali emergency relief, and (3) as competitive supplier—as in the case of the Australian Passport Information Service.
6   It is clear that the Government came to realize it could not contract out public income support service provision to private providers.

9
Getting to Count: The Looking After Children (LAC) Initiative

Anna Yeatman and Joanna Penglase

You know you cannot take for granted that just because a child comes into care, this is going to make things better. [There has been] a considerable shift over the last couple of decades in out of home care. There was an assumption that if you took a child into care and because they were having a problem at home, that you … were doing them a great favour. Longitudinal research is telling us [this is not so]. So LAC is … designed to ask … you to review things at set places. It's asking you to include people who know the child best. And this is quite revolutionary you know. … it really confronts people, this sharing of information … [T]here's little revolutions going on all over the place because of LAC … When it's used as it's intended, it actually gets people talking together who … are not routinely [involved]. Oftentimes, parents and carers, and even the child themselves, are excluded from care planning … And so plans often times fail… [There] is no point sending this child to this particular school, they went there two years ago, they had a really bad run, it's the same principal, this is setting this child up to fail … Now if [the worker does] not have this information … they may have the best of intentions … but when you're making decisions around care planning you need to include the people who know the child best (Jude Morwitzer, Program Manager, The LAC Project Australia, interview data, Sydney, March 2003).

Introduction

Historically, children in 'out-of-home' care have been at risk of institutional neglect, abuse, and abandonment in ways that tragically compound the difficulties they may have experienced in their family of

141

origin. In context of a general shift away from institutional to community based services, children and young people who are administratively assessed as needing out-of-home care services are today placed mostly in foster or kin care settings.

A number of factors have combined to create an impetus for a systemic approach to individualized care planning for children and young people who need out-of-home care. Firstly, now children and young people, rhetorically at least, are accepted as persons to whom contemporary standards of human rights and inclusion in decision making process should apply. Secondly, it is a well accepted fact that, historically, the administrative practice of statutory government departments charged with handling the cases of children deemed to need out-of-home care has been crisis-oriented and unsystematic. An administrative environment that is chronically understaffed, overworked, where there is high worker turn-over, makes it difficult for the individual case to be handled in a continuous manner by the one worker or single team of workers. If there are no continuous and readily retrievable records regarding the individual in care, it is impossible for there to be effective monitoring of their progression through time or timely response to problems in care experienced by the individual. These individuals 'get lost in the system', there is a lack of coordination across the various agencies involved with the individual, and positive policy statements are not matched by practice (Cashmore, Dolby and Brennan 1994, 42). Cashmore, Dolby and Brennan (1994, 10) call this 'systems abuse', defining this as abuse that is 'perpetuated not by a single person or agency, but by the entire child care system stretched beyond its limits'. Thirdly, and partly related to such administrative 'systems abuse', young people who have been in the care system are less likely than other young people to complete their secondary education and gain employment, and are at greater risk of homelessness, poverty, mental health problems, substance abuse, involvement in crime and teenage parenthood (Cashmore and Ainsworth 2004, 27; see also Mendes and Moslehuddin 2004).

In this case study, we discuss the Looking After Children (LAC) initiative first in general and then with reference to its adoption by Barnardos in Australia. LAC is an administrative tool for service planning and systematic process (Austin and McLelland 1996) in the management of individual cases that is intended to make front-line social work practice in the area of out-of-home care informed by current research, accountable, transparent, integrated, continuous, and stakeholder responsive. LAC is intended to create a rational and transparent link between process and outcomes (Jackson 1998, 54). Without process and procedure that make it possible to record, track and link decisions concerning a child or young person in care, it is impossible to hold those who are responsible for the management of this individual's 'case' responsible, let alone facilitate practice that carefully, respectfully, and practically attends to the child/young person's needs and, so far as it may be possible, wants. The advocates of LAC do not see it as a panacea (Roy Parker 1998, 20). How could it be in a welfare area that is associated with the needs of individuals who do not have the right to vote, does not attract political interest in reform, and where the statutory agency responsible for the handling of children in care 'has a low political profile' (Cashmore, Dolby and Brennan 1994, 36) because its clients are poor and stigmatized and its workers lowly paid and largely female (Hasenfeld 1992, especially 7–9)? LAC is best regarded as an individualized and integrated information system (Steyaert 1997, 13) that can facilitate better management of individuals and bring to light system failure that can be rectified.

Professional advocacy of individualization in the delivery of welfare services is often responsible for important innovation in both frontline service work and policy; it is professionals (primarily social workers) that have been the advocates for the adoption of the LAC framework for guiding practice. Their advocacy is to be seen in context of a complex social process of coming to terms with historically entrenched patterns of what is now called child abuse, a process that has increased the volume of demand on the out-of-home care system as well as created opportunities for a populist media in exploiting an atmosphere of crisis that attends well-publicized cases of horrific abuse of children. Thus the demand for reform of systems comes at a time when the out of care system is under terrific pressure which may only get worse. Consider in this connection these propositions offered by Cashmore and Ainsworth (2004, 13), two respected child welfare researchers in Australia:

> Child welfare services are under severe pressure in every state in Australia, in the US and the UK as increasing numbers of children are coming to the notice of the statutory child protection authorities. The number of children in out-of-home care has increased each year since 1996 when there were 13,979 children in out-of-home care, an overall increase of 45% ... The most recent Australian figures indicate that there were 20,297 children in out-of-home care in Australia as at 30 June 2003. The rate for Indigenous children in

out-of-home care is nearly seven times the rate for non-Indigenous children.

The increasing demand comes at a time when the supply of foster carers and professionally trained and experienced workers is under increasing pressure. Most children entering care (91%) are in some form of foster care ... although it is increasingly clear that other options are needed for the growing numbers who enter care with serious problems ...

While state governments are committing increased resources especially to child protection investigation, more resources by themselves will not resolve the problem. All too readily extra resources simply lead to more of the same, and it is by no means clear that what is being done for children is producing positive outcomes. Alongside these extra resources, a research-led reform strategy is needed to support the next generation of evidence-based child welfare policy and service developments.

Out-of-home care is a complex area of welfare service provision because it involves children and young people who still need parental care and love, whose own parents have been unable to provide this on a sustained basis, who may have ongoing ties to their parents, but who are also positioned in a set of relationships to an administrative system, one or more case workers, and foster parents. The stakeholders

Table 9.1   Features of institutions that facilitate systems abuse
(from Cashmore, Dolby and Brennan 1994, 36)

Arising from particular political and administrative decisions
1. Lack of resources
2. Gap between policy and practice
3. Lack of coordination and consistency
4. Inadequate guidelines
5. Lack of specialized skills
6. Lack of support for staff
7. Lack of information
8. Lack of a voice for children

Arising from the features of bureaucracies
9. System for the system's sake
10. Structural insulation

are multiple, some of them with complex investments in the child or young person, there is a child or young person who has a difficult and possibly traumatic family history, there is a risk-averse administrative system, and an under-resourced welfare sector.

If we examine Table 9.1 'Features of institutions that facilitate systems abuse', it is clear that LAC as such can do nothing about factors 1 (lack of resources), 2 (gap between policy and practice), 9 and 10, but that it can do something about factors 3, 4, 5, 6, 7 and 8, and in so doing, it may make the issues regarding factors 1, 2, 9 and 10 more visible.

Development and take up of LAC across national jurisdictions

LAC was first initiated in the United Kingdom. The LAC materials were published in 1995 and promoted by the Department of Health following the development of these materials and a long process of consultation around them (Parker 1998; Bell 1998/1999; Jackson 1998). The approach and the materials were driven by professionals who had experience and expertise in the area and who found in the Department of Health an administrative champion. The materials have been widely adopted throughout Britain by local authorities as their *modus operandi* for the substitute care system for children (Jackson 1998).

LAC has been taken up in other countries such as Sweden, Canada and Australia (Jones, Clark, Kufeldt and Norrman 1998, 215). The take up is varied in the degree to which the full LAC system is adopted as distinct from just the LAC Assessment and Action records. As reported in 2004, Canadian provinces were using just the latter (The LAC Project Australia *Newsletter*, March 2004, no pagination), whereas in Australia, where LAC has been adopted, it is the full system that is used.

In Australia take-up has been by state governments in Victoria, Australian Capital Territory, Tasmania and Western Australia (Tregeagle and Treleaven 2006, 360), which is the level of government that has responsibility for statutory welfare work with children. In New South Wales, the most populous state, a non-government organization dedicated to advocacy for children—Barnardos Australia—is working with the University of New South Wales as the Australian-licensed promoter of UK-developed LAC materials. LAC is now normal Barnardos practice in working with children who need out-of-home care. As of August 2004, 20% of children in care in NSW were care managed by agencies using LAC (The LAC Project Australia *Newsletter*, August 2004, no pagination). The statutory department in NSW (Department of

Community Services, DoCS) does not use LAC. At the same time the NSW Office of the Children's Guardian has developed an Accreditation and Quality Improvement Program which under the Children and Young Persons (Care and Protection) Act 1998 requires all organizations (including the statutory department) providing out-of-home care to be accredited. Barnardos Australia was the first agency to be accredited. DoCS, the statutory agency, is participating in the accreditation and quality improvement program and, according to its *Annual Review 2005/2006* (52), it is 'on track to receive full accreditation before the legislated deadline of July 2013'. This may prompt the state-wide adoption of LAC as the systemic approach to care planning and management.

Barnardos Australia developed LACES, the electronic version of LAC to support the Australian adaptation of the LAC system. LAC was conceived in such a way that a computer-based information system developed around each child could be integrated with the aggregate collection of data by the government agency responsible for policy and program development in this area of welfare services (see Steyaert 1997).[1] In Australia, Tasmania was the first State government to implement LACS as a whole system using LACES (computer based recording) (The LAC Project Australia *Newsletter March 2004*, no pagination). Unlike the United Kingdom, however, there is no national information system for children in care in Australia primarily because historically responsibility in this area has been handled by State governments. The lack of a national strategy for research, data gathering and policy development limits the possibilities of effective policy learning in this area. Children's advocates (Tregeagle and Treleaven 2006, 360; Cashmore and Ainsworth 2004) regard this as a major problem. Cashmore and Ainsworth (2004, 45) comment:

> ... there is no systematic approach to research in relation to out-of-home care in Australia. There is urgent need for a research and development strategy for [this] ... sector. There is no national research agenda and most state departments have yet to develop a research agenda to inform their core business or are only now beginning to do so.

Our fieldwork

In the following discussion, as well as referring to the academic and promotional literature on LAC, we are drawing upon fieldwork data based on several interviews conducted in Sydney in the period from the end of 2002 to early 2003. Barnardos Australia has been the non-

government agency that has created The LAC Project, a business initiative where it is licensed by the UK parent program to promote the
program and train workers to use it. Barnardos has also adopted LAC as
its approach to children in both short-term (under ten months) and
long-term care. Through Barnardos in Sydney, we got access to the
LAC forms and related operational print material. We interviewed both
the senior manager and the program manager for the LAC Project.[2] We
also interviewed two Barnardos case workers and a LAC team leader all
involved in the early stages of introducing this new approach into clinical practice. We observed a discussion conducted by four of this
agency's caseworkers on aspects of LAC practice. We interviewed one
young person involved in the program, his foster carer and the foster
carer of one other young person. Our work in the field occurred when
LAC was being first implemented in Australia and before its take-up
had become as comprehensive as it has now become. This chapter in
draft has been factually corrected by Jude Morwitzer, the Program
Manager of the Barnardos LAC Project.

Describing LAC

The Looking After Children materials underpin a case management
approach to care assessment, planning and review for children in out-of-
home care, developed by the UK Department of Health over a period of
several years from 1987 (Wise 2003, 39) in collaboration with academic
advisers who built into the approach a reliance on current knowledge
about children and their developmental needs. 'The materials comprise a
comprehensive system of information gathering, planning and review
documents' (Bell 1998/1999, 15). Deidre Dixon (now Deidre Cheers), the
Australian LAC Project Senior Manager, provides this overall description
of LAC:

> LAC is a guided practice case management system requiring in-
> formation about a child in care to be collected in a standardised
> way. It generates a best practice approach to planning, decision
> making, reviewing and monitoring for children in out-of-home care.
> LAC is about engaging with key people, most particularly the child
> and his/her parents, and those who are providing the direct day-to-
> day care—foster parents and direct carers (Dixon 2001, 27).

LAC creates an individualized and documented planning trail around
each child in care (Clarke and Burke 1998, 2–3; Clare 1997, 32–33). The

trail is articulated as a client information system (Steyaert 1997) that has both paper and electronic recording aspects.

The LAC client information system consists of two kinds of forms— The first set of forms frame the key points of service planning: entry into the service, assessment, service review, and service exit. The service planning forms are: the *Essential Information Record*, the *Care Plan*, the *Placement Plan* and the *Review of Arrangements*. These forms, each having a different colour to distinguish their different function, provide for description of the child in terms of individual needs and characteristics, and then track this information into an individualized care and placement plan. As the senior manager, The LAC project, put it to us, 'it separates out the nitty-gritty day to day of the child's life, from the big-picture of why they're actually in care'. The *Essential Information Record* is therefore divided into two parts. Part 1 gives information needed immediately by carers, Part 2 presents a comprehensive description of the child's background, legal status, and placement history. The *Placement Plan* also is divided into two. Part 1 carries the agreement for the child to be looked after, with a record of essential names and addresses, while Part 2 contains more detailed information of the child's world—everyday routines, social and leisure activities—as well as covering health, education, identity and access issues. The *Care Plan* describes what the child needs in a placement, and the strategy for achieving this. Regardless of how many siblings are being placed, each child has his/her own set of forms. The *Review of Arrangements* is used to document the decisions that are made at the points of mandatory review that are built into the LAC process of service planning. A *Review of Arrangements* is conducted within one month of placement, then at intervals of four months after placement, then ten months after placement, and, if the child continues in care, at six-monthly intervals.

Secondly, the more controversial and elaborate set of forms called the Assessment and Action Records (AARs) are age-related records that set 'specific age-related objectives for children's progress (Ward 1998, 207)'. While both sets of forms are 'guided' by direct and explicit reference in the left-hand margin to evidence-based 'best practice', this is especially the case with the AARs. For example in the AAR form for children aged one and two years (this is the LAC form provided to us by Barnardos-Australia, adapted for use in Australia), there is a question 'How frequently is the child read to, shown picture books or shown stories?' with boxes next to it to tick for the most appropriate answer ('daily', 'some days only', 'once a week or less', 'don't know', and so on). In the left margin the best practice note reads: 'Reading to very young children is important as it helps to develop their knowledge and understanding of words and language; as well as increasing their familiarity with books and an interest in them.' The AARs are designed to cover the developmental stages of children and young people. In their bulk and scope they are formidable. In total, the AARs constitute six sets of age-related records covering the same seven developmental dimensions. They require those using the forms to answer questions that are designed both to measure progress for an individual child/young person and to determine whether this individual is getting the assistance s/he may need to progress. For children under one year, 35 pages of information are required to be filled out (this would be coordinated by the case worker in relation to the carer and appropriate others) and close to 60 pages for those aged 15 or over (this would be filled out by the young person herself with the assistance of the most appropriate adult). The first is to be completed within ten months of placement and then annually if the child is over five years, six monthly if less than age five (Clare 1997, 32–33; Barnardos LAC Flowchart).

In sum, LAC is an individualized planning tool which gives both a systematic and reflexive aspect to the process of service delivery. All advocates of LAC emphasize that LAC in use can live up to the promise of its design only if it used by creative, skilled social workers. This design of LAC permits:

- care planning to be individualized—that is centred on the individual child
- the engagement of all primary stakeholders in the process
- a systematic recording of information
- the ready accessibility of these records
- the tracking over time of a child's career through the care system
- the accountability of all persons involved in the child's care, and
- the monitoring and review of a child's case in the care system.

The core assumption underpinning LAC is that good, transparent, accountable and inclusive process is the necessary though not sufficient means by which better outcomes for children in out-of-home care can be produced by those responsible for the public management and front-line delivery of such care.

The Barnardos Australia LAC Project

Barnardos Australia, headquartered in Sydney, is a 'non-government child welfare agency which provides support and care services for children and families, (Dixon 2001, 28) in both New South Wales and the Australian Capital Territory. In 1997, in consortium with the School of Social Work, University of New South Wales, Barnardos Australia established 'The LAC Project Australia'. 'By January 1998 there was full implementation of the LAC system (Planning, Placement, and Review materials as well as Assessment and Action Records) in all Barnardos out-of-home care teams' (Dixon and Morwitzer 2001, 3).

Operationally in relation to government and other non-government agencies, Barnardos Australia has been the lead agency in promoting the LAC approach: 'we applied to Britain for a commercial license which would then allow us' 'to impact on the lives of all children [in Australia], not just children in NSW and the ACT',[3] 'and on-sell the system' (from interview with Deidre Dixon 2001). It is not a commercial business in the sense of profit orientation:

> The agreement between Barnardos and the University I think is that any money generated goes back into the development of the project. And the price [of materials etc] is to cover costs. ... the reason we did it that way was basically because of the [Barnardos] Board's commitment to wanting to change children's lives, rather than to make money (from interview with Deidre Dixon 2001).

By the time we interviewed the LAC Project senior manager and program manager (in 2001, and 2002), they had several years experience of implementing LAC within Barnardos out-of-home care services and of introducing it in other agencies and government systems. We thus report first on how they understood this implementation experience.

In Barnardos Australia practice, LAC applies only where children have been placed with non-related persons. In addition, the majority of children and young people are placed in short-term care (for ten months or under), and for short-term placements, the service planning forms rather than the AARs are used (according to our interview with the LAC Program Manager).

The LAC flow chart used by Barnardos Australia outlines unequivocally the expected time periods in which events are to occur. The administration of all the care planning forms is anchored to a timeline which is specified. There are also designated requirements for signing off for the forms that frame the large decision points in a child's career through care. Workers are trained to use the forms appropriately and under supervision provided by their immediate manager. In use, these forms lay out the pathways for the service planning process and provide the checkpoints where the worker in dialogue with the child and his/her carer and maybe also his/her parent of origin are to discuss and decide on key issues (schooling for example). Accordingly it is in how the worker uses the forms that they provide structure and focus for service planning and the process of interaction it actually involves.

Implementation lessons and insights

The LAC Project senior manager has emphasized the importance of strong and committed leadership, a careful and planned organizational change strategy, the development of an inclusive team management approach to changing front-line practice, the provision of professional supervision of LAC in use, and a named Project Leader, as key components of successful implementation of the LAC approach in front-line agency practice (see Dixon 2001; Dixon and Morwitzer 2001). Essentially the emphasis is on a long-term approach to embedding LAC as normal social work practice within the agency's *modus operandi*, and the focus is on LAC in use with attention given to a management practice where workers are trained, skilled, monitored and supervised in using this approach.

Early on in the implementation of LAC in Barnardos, the difficulty of reconciling 'busy caseloads' with the establishment work and learning involved in adopting a new care system was recognized; the CEO of Barnardos gave the instruction that, 'if required, caseloads were to be dropped and additional resources brought in (from interview with Jude Morwitzer, Barnardos Project Leader March 2003)'. Dixon (2001, 31) comments on the same issue in relation to a study of factors affecting LAC implementation in Barnardos in the first year:

> ... program size had an effect on the use of LAC in Barnardos. Four of the five teams with 100% compliance supervised less than twenty children in care. Having fewer forms requiring completion for low numbers in care, and thus making it easier for the manager to track implementation meant that the smaller programs showed increased compliance to LAC in Barnardos.

Jude Morwitzer, the LAC Project manager in Barnardos told us that Barnardos has been an agency that has regarded itself as leading best practice in child welfare work, but that with the introduction of LAC, the issue of whether rhetoric was matched by reality became highly visible. Precisely for this reason, she stressed the importance of careful change management process and appropriate support for and skilling of front-line workers: 'your workers need to know what it is, why they're bringing it in, and they need to know what LAC replaces (interview with Jude Morwitzer, March 2003)'. Here are a number of her reflections on the implementation of LAC where she is indicating how it has provoked discussion among those involved in this process:

> What we learnt is that LAC is very insidious. It actually infiltrates a program in ways people never thought it would. It provokes discussions about who you actually recruit as carers ... Because if you're saying that carers [are to be included] and they're handling confidential information ... you need to be recruiting carers that you believe have the capacity ... to handle confidential information, with training.

> ... by and large people at Barnardos thought that they belonged to an agency that was a best practice agency. ... [I]t has been confronting. ... it makes things so transparent ... are you really doing this? Or are you just saying you're doing this? How do I know that the young person has participated? Well, I gave them a copy and that. But how is that participation? So there's been a lot of discussion about what is participation?

> [I]n Barnardos there is, by and large, very good supervision systems ... Most workers would be seen once a month ... at least for a two-hour period ... to look at their casework and how they're doing. ... Team leaders ... comment that it's [LAC] helpful ... It's a much longer implementation phase that I ever would have expected. Because ... it confronts people so much and it goes through every part of your systems ... It's not just case management, it's the carer recruitment, it's the carer training in induction, it's the basic premise on how you operate around handling information across the board, with anybody. You know, how you interact with other agencies, they're a non-LAC agency, we're a LAC agency; do I give them the LAC records? Why wouldn't you give them the LAC records? I don't usually give them our files ... It sparks questions and discussions ... about so many issues.

> I think the issues of feedback from young people have been neglected ... because it's complex to do. ... Also when you're chan-

ging a system, you actually ... need to get it in place first ... So that
the young people ... aren't victims of an agency learning how to
do something ... It's still very early days with LAC. I mean, we're
five years down the track ...

These statements are indicative not just of a coherent and sustained
leadership from this agency in developing social work practice so that
it could underpin LAC in use, but also of the real time perspective that
needs to be adopted in relation to embedding a transparent, accountable, stakeholder inclusive and reflective approach in service planning.
It is not just that LAC represents an historic change in the ethos of
service planning—making it more explicit, accountable, transparent
and participatory.[4] It is also that good practice can never be taken for
granted. It has to be planned for, led, managed, supported, supervised
and resourced on an ongoing basis. In this respect, this case study
confirms what we learnt from the case study of employment services
for people with a psychiatric disability (see Chapter 12). Considered
simply as an individualized service planning technology LAC achieves
nothing—its value in use has entirely to do with the intention, quality,
judgement and skill of those who put it into practice. As Dixon and
Morwitzer (2001, 7) contend: 'Using LAC in the way it is intended
requires thought and a commitment to an inclusive style of working.'
Intentional use of an evidence-based approach to good service practice
is a value commitment. It depends on a clear enunciation and understanding of the values that are to inform and guide good practice.
    We turn now to some of the features of LAC that make it similar
to the employment service planning process discussed in Chapter 12:
firstly, the aspect of service planning that involves signing off and
review, and how this underwrites the values of accountability and
transparency; secondly, the emphasis in the LAC approach to the
creation of a service planning record that is integrated with a best practice approach to the service in question; and finally, the inclusive and
participatory aspect of this service planning approach.

Signing off and review—the values of accountability and transparency

In concluding (2001, 8) paper, Dixon and Morwitzer say, 'Yes, LAC brings
with it increased scrutiny and accountability, but more importantly it
shares the power and the "sign off" of plans, which not everyone feels
comfortable with or likes'. *As service planning*, LAC is structured as a set

of explicit and recorded decision nodes. In the case of the 'Placement Plan', its last page is headed 'This plan has been discussed with the following, who agree to its provisions'. Then follows boxes for name, signature and date for each of: the child/young person, mother, father, other (please identify), foster carer/residential worker, case worker, and supervisor. Then follows a section: 'Please note areas of disagreement.' The 'Review of Arrangements' document includes a consultation and assessment section where the case worker is to enter information prior to the review about whether she has discussed 'what should be considered at this review' with the child/young person, his/her mother, his/her father, his/her carer(s), the independent visitor, any other interested person; there is a record of the people invited to the review; a record of discussion which is guided by a checklist of issues to consider; a section asking for confirmation that the child, parents, foster carers have been advised of their rights to appeal and case review; and concludes with space for signing off by the review chair, statutory officer if relevant, and caseworker with, finally, a list of boxes to be ticked, confirming a copy of this document has been sent to: the child/young person, his/her mother, his/her father, other adult(s) with parental responsibility, carer(s), other review participants (if applicable), and other persons consulted before the review (if applicable).

As an individual or personal record of a child's history in care, LAC functions in two time frameworks. We refer to the Assessment and Action records: first, they operate in a present-future oriented temporality where they are intended as a set of prompts for the young person or, if too young to do this himself, for someone acting on his behalf, to scope and review their needs across seven developmental dimensions in order to prompt action if necessary. Second, they offer a retrospective personal history for the young person. The back of the record includes a tabular summary of plans for action—'work required', 'persons responsible', 'target date', 'date completed', and 'decisions about actions that are desirable but cannot happen yet'—that matches up with assessment sections within the AAR. For example in the AAR for children aged ten to 14 years, under 'What do you hope to be doing in three years time?', there is a further question, 'Would you like any help and advice about making plans for the future? If so who will give this to you?', after which follows the prompt, 'Please record details about plans for further action and target dates in the summary at the back of this Record.'

As with the employment plans discussed in Chapter 12, the explicit recording of decisions taken, of who has said they will do what, and of their 'signing off', with provision for periodic review, injects into LAC a form of relational contracting. This is the aspect of signing off that the case worker we interviewed emphasized in discussing the LAC Care Plan:

> ... it's [the Care Plan] like a contract. So, if you don't sign a contract, then it's not, you know. So ... if you didn't get the [statutory] Department say to sign it, or the child to sign it ... and then later down the track if there's a decision ... that the Department's to pay private school fees ... and if it's not signed, you go back later to get the school fees and they say, we never signed that.

Review of Care Plans occur at stipulated intervals, and these provide the mechanism for determining whether the decisions that have been agreed to have actually been carried out by those who committed to undertake them. The same case worker who had only recently started working at Barnardos after having worked for the statutory department for three years made an interesting point of contrast between the two care planning practices. With LAC, those who sign off indicate they have done so by name in contrast to the statutory department:

> I've found that they [the statutory department] don't do that. ... I did put task ... [and] use names, and my supervisor said no, don't use names, take the name away, and just put 'caseworker' ... I don't know, maybe it's because the turnover of staff may be more frequent ...

She said also regarding the same contrast that the statutory department did not have a procedure for review:

> ... the Department doesn't have a procedure, so it's just whatever everyone thinks, when shall we have the next review? And then that may be written on the minutes of a meeting or something, but then not followed through because something else has come up, and they've cancelled that meeting, and then it's not followed through. Where LAC helps you follow through, you know, you've got to have the meeting, there's no question about it ... And if it's cancelled ... which was for me last week ... [due to] unforeseeable circumstances of the young person ... another meeting has to be followed through. You know, it has to be done. It's just the procedure and the way we do it. But there's no set ... rule for the Department ... just an individual management ... decision ... And it may be because they don't have the time ... and then its other priorities take place ...

An integrated client information system

LAC is a carefully designed client information system that allows the information needs of managers and policy makers to be embedded into an information system that also addresses the information needs of the service provider (Steyaert 1997, 13), and that is maintained over time. LAC is also an information system that addresses the need of the young person to have a personal record of their stay in care: the Assessment and Action records are regarded as the property of the young person. Deidre Dixon, in interview with us, comments on this aspect of the LAC information system, and in a moment we shall see why this is so important:

> ... in practice what we do [and suggest to] other agencies is that if the young person doesn't want to keep the original document themselves, that they keep those original documents as a separate set ... rather than as a routine part of the file. And if the young person or child takes the original copy of the document that they keep a copy.

A key goal of LAC is to create a 'corporate parent' who 'pays attention to the details of a child's lived experience, just as biological parents do (Dixon 2001, 27)'. In our interview with her, Deidre Dixon explained what this phrase 'corporate parent' meant:

> The 'corporate parent' is ... multiple people. So it's the child for whom perhaps with a legal order, but not necessarily, someone has made a decision, and for a voluntary placement it might be a parent saying 'Barnardos, would you look after my child for two weeks?' So they sign a placement agreement and the carer signs the placement agreement and the worker signs the placement agreement and they all agree that this is what they're going to do for that two weeks. As soon as that's done, besides that parent, you have the direct care social worker. You might have a foster mother and/or a foster father and/or adult children and/or other children in the household. You might have a different doctor because the carer, if the child gets sick, might involve her own GP as opposed to the one the child has gone to. If the child is placed in an area that is not close to home they might move school. So you immediately expand the number of people who are having a say in that child's life. And that's the corporate parent—the idea that there are multiple people involved.

She commented further of the corporate parent that it is 'potentially huge' which is why the guided aspect of the LAC information system is so important: 'it actually specifies ... who does and who doesn't have access to information'. She continues:

> So that if you don't have to have the information you don't get it. Direct carers and parents always get it and it puts decision-making and practice into the realms of more public accountability if you like. So it takes away from a social worker sitting in an office making a decision that really and truly you know, Johnny should go to this school and not that one. And then having the personal debate if you like with the carer who says 'no, no, but his friends are there, I want him to go there.' Invariably ... the social worker will [have] more of a say than the direct carer.

Of disagreement she said: 'our expectation and our practice experience would be that just the fact of having this system ... decreases the opportunity for that level of disagreement', and if it occurs, it is recorded.

LAC, then, works with the reality of what is a fact of life for most children in out-of-home care, particularly children who remain in care over a considerable period of time: that they are unlikely to have only one caseworker in that period, likely indeed to have several, as well as a number of other key people involved in their lives at any one time. In accepting this reality, the LAC approach can work with it. Knowledge about a child in care is held by a large number of people who are not necessarily in communication with each other and who may change, sometimes quite often. Many of these people will disappear from the child's life, along with their information about the child, which may be in their head, or recorded where it is not easily found. As the Program Manager for the LAC project told us in our interview with her:

> [LAC] keeps track of all those bits and pieces of information that, for children living with their own families, their own parent carries around in their head. Children in the care system, you know they're lucky if someone carries it for them and that person stays long enough to actually remember that they had measles when they were two.

> [LAC] has well-developed communication systems [both] ... in time and over time. ... [I]t's not as dependent upon any one person being there for that life, because it reflects the fact that people are changing constantly ... If you didn't have people changing constantly you wouldn't need to write things down as much. ... [It is] a very structured system in that certain sorts of knowledges [sic] are held in certain sorts of records. So if you wanted to know

particular pieces of information or check back what had been previous ... there are very predictable places you put information.
So this means, not only is knowledge recorded, it's actually accessible ... accessibility is an important factor ... you need to have
information held in ways that it can be drawn out again for use.

People see paper and people see forms ... and it's very hard to see
that this ... actually forms part of a living process ... [I]t's an integral
part to be able to work towards outcomes ... writing things down.
So I usually start [a] presentation [on LAC] with ... LAC uses this
wonderful technology ..., this marvellous communication tool
which allows me to speak to somebody ... now at this time, or
to hear this child then years ago or ten years in the future. ... It's
called writing. And I said, until we have something better, writing
still is the most reliable communication source that we currently
have. And writing things down, in places where you know the
information is kept, is the next best step too.

It is also intended to provide a child or young person with a record
of their time in care. The value of a continuous and readily retrievable
record of one's individual history in care is something that is clear to
Joanna Penglase (one of this chapter's authors) because of her experience
as someone who spent their childhood in a children's home. For people
who have grown up with their parents, there is usually ready access to
photographs, family stories, and mementoes that provide a living record
of their place as an individual in their family history; and if their parents
are still living, these individuals can ask the kinds of reflective questions
an adult might ask about why did that happen, why did you send me
to that school, and so on. Joanna Penglase (2005, 322–326) documents a
time when record keeping about children in care was not a high priority
with either the statutory agency or the charitable sector, a time when
generally adult authorities explained nothing to children especially if they
were children in care (see Penglase 2005, 266–269). Where the records
were kept, the information is impersonal and judgemental (Penglase
2005, 323), and often they were not kept at all. The importance of a record
keeping system that integrates the different needs for information—the
system's, the service agency's, and the individual's 'personal' perspective—can be readily overlooked if it is not understood that this may be
the only information resource an individual has to find out about their
childhood history. Of people who were not state wards the statutory
department kept no individual information. Penglase (2005, 324) says of

this: 'I, for example, did not exist for the NSW Department in a personal file, and this is the case for all children growing up in non-government Homes.' She continues:

> What non-wards get from their [Home] varies greatly; when they do manage to get their records, they generally find that there is almost nothing written in the file about them, sometimes for their entire childhoods. Often they appear on an admission and a discharge register, with nothing at all in between. Details of parents and siblings, and the reasons children have come into care, are not always recorded; and sometimes birthdays and other details are actually incorrect. It can be almost guaranteed that nothing will be written about their development or individual characteristics—there will be nothing personal at all.

In this context the significance of two distinct comments on the LAC information system becomes clear. The first is that of Jude Morwitzer, the LAC Program Manager:

> … where there is disagreement there is room on the LAC records for them to note their disagreement. And that's important to know too. You know, kids will often say, you know, why didn't mum, why did mum want me to … ? And there in black and white is, mum didn't want to, mum felt she had to.

The second is that of a highly valued Barnardos male carer, valued because he has accepted the role of foster carer of three male siblings who prior to this point had a traumatic and abusive history with another foster carer. The three boys 'placed themselves' with this man because of knowing him through their relationship to his sons. We interviewed this foster carer and the middle boy who was 15 at this time. His carer first expressed very little patience with what he saw as bureaucratic form filling that could not possibly match they constantly changing complexities of these boys' lives; he also was protective of them, doubting that written down information that keeps a record of behaviour that later the individual may be shamed by could be a good thing; and then, in dialogue with Joanna Penglase, his interviewer, there is a shift in his perception:

> *Foster* carer: Oh God … I'd never seen so many forms … I dunno if it's a good thing … because things change so quickly with

them ... it's very personal ... it's like making a record of your life and ... the questions that are being asked ... and someone can get these ... 20 years down the track, and say, well you know, you used to do this and you used to that, and you was an alcoholic, and you were a drug addict and all of this. And I've got the proof ...

Interviewer: ... it enables them to have a record of their childhood. Which a lot of kids in care don't have, you know, often they don't even know where they were.

Foster carer: Yeah, that's why I think it's a good idea.

Interviewer: ... they get a copy and it's there if they want it. So ten years down the track if they think, well, what was that all about, that period of my life, at least they can open it up and there it is. That's the thinking behind it.

Foster carer: Yeah ... I s'pose so. [Pause]

Interviewer: But you feel you've got reservations ...

Foster carer: ... yeah, I'm thinking, not being a ward myself, knowing, oh well I suppose I have my mum and dad to go back to if I need questions asked. Mmm.

The inclusive and participatory character of the LAC service planning approach

LAC is designed to keep the process centred on the needs and wants of the individual child and to involve all ground level stakeholders in discussion and decision about the child's care. The commitment to stakeholder involvement is exemplified in the *Care Plan* which is the 'big picture' of why the child is in care. As detailed above, an entire page is given to the sign-off process, beginning with the statement that 'this plan has been discussed with the following who have recorded whether or not they agree', and followed by the recording of the signatures of the child/young person, the mother, father, other(s) with parental responsibility, foster carer/residential care worker, other interested relative (if applicable), case worker, manager/supervisor, and statutory authority delegated officer. If any of those listed have not been consulted, the following section provides a large space in which to explain why. Further, the remaining space requests details if any of those listed disagree with any provision of the plan.

The *Review of Arrangements* comes with a set of *Consultation Papers*, one each for the child/young person, the direct carer, and the parent/parental figure. Each carries a set of questions which can be used as a prompt for reflection about issues to be raised. All relevant stakeholders may be present at reviews, including the parent(s) where possible and appropriate. The forms can be used to record opinions by stakeholders who either cannot or choose not to attend the meeting. However not all stakeholders are accorded the same priority of status: the *Consultation Paper* for carers assumes their presence at a review meeting but those for the child/young person and the parent simply urge that 'you should come to your (your child's) review if you possibly can'. Where a stakeholder chooses not to attend, their completed copy of the Consultation Paper should be sent to the meeting so that their views can be taken into account and recorded.

In interview with the LAC Program Manager, Jude Morwitzer, she confirmed the observation made by others that the birth parents are not as readily included as the foster carer: 'Carers get the first inclusion, usually, then, the young person, and then parents, in terms of hierarchy of inclusion'. In part this reflects the LAC programmatic emphasis on a collaborative partnership between case worker and foster carer, and it also reflects the complexities surrounding the inclusion of birth parents who for some reason are not in a position to assume the parental role in relation to their child.

LAC builds in the participation and voice of the child/young person. The 'form filling' aspect of LAC has attracted criticism (discussed by Yeatman and Penglase 2004, 242–243). As we discovered with the foster carer and young person we talked to in Sydney these forms can be perceived as serving bureaucratic rather than the child or young person's needs where the young person will say anything to the worker 'just to get the question over and done with' (according to the foster carer). In this case it is only fair to add that the LAC approach had only just been introduced to these two individuals by a Barnardos case worker still learning the LAC ropes. However, this case worker, whom we interviewed after saying that she found the AARs 'very tedious', indicated a more complex perspective when she said it prompted having a conversation with the young person that she would not otherwise have had. Her comments confirm what the literature has reported, still scantily because the implementation of LAC in the UK, Australia, Canada and elsewhere is still in process of being analysed, that some young people find filling out the AARs valuable: 'it looked at other issues in my life that no-one had ever talked to me about before', and 'This gives us time to think and say what we really want (Bernice quoted by Kearns with Bernice and Margaret 1996, 86)'. The case worker we interviewed had this to say:

> [I]t's a very adult-centric world ... Even though we are becoming a lot more informed and trying to ... better our practices and follow the UN Convention on the rights of the children by giving them a voice and getting them to participate in decision-making ... we've still got a long way to go. Especially with younger children ... we still don't understand them. ... LAC doesn't really ... solve all the problems ... this helps children have a voice ... Whether or not it actually changes things, it hears them and things are recorded.

Jude Morwitzer, the LAC Program Manager, in our interview with her, described how one young person, who was keen to participate in her care decisions but who did not like going to the review meetings, managed her participation. This young girl told her:

> My worker always comes out and talks to me before they go to review meetings, and takes notes about what I think 's important, and should happen, and I trust that she tells because I also get a copy of the Minutes, so I know she's said it because it's in the Minutes. And I also get to see what other people said, and I also get to see what were the decisions so I can know what's supposed to happen for me.

Jude Morwitzer went on to offer a set of reflections which indicate the complex and relational nature of the engagement of the child or young person in participation in their care service. We include the interviewer's questions:

> *Interviewer*: So how important is the young person's voice in their care?

> *JM*: Look it's absolutely crucial. Communication's an extraordinarily complex thing. And workers are asked to make judgments all the time about things...and some of the time they're real shots in the

dark ... [I]f the sole aim is to ... assist with life outcomes for the young person you can't do this without including the young person ... The skill comes in ... setting up processes for participation that are age appropriate ... and ... include a young person in a way that has meaning for them ... For some young people, like that young girl, it may mean never going to a meeting. For some people, it will mean going to a meeting. For some young people it'll mean being very overtly included in meetings from quite a young age, which means you'll have to change your usual meeting structure because they can't sit there for two hours ...

Interviewer: Do you think there are difficulties in children being taken seriously, having a voice?

JM: Oh, huge difficulties, Joanna.

Interviewer: What are they?

JM: People make assumptions that children don't know ... People then say they wish children to participate and they wish to listen, but they set the process up in a way that it's counter-productive to there being any meaningful participation. ... You've actually got to ... take the time to ... pick what does [a child mean] ... Like, I never want to see Mum again ... And then when you say, well how long did you live with Mum? And how long have you been in care, did you write your Mum letters? Did you telephone your Mum ... that thoughtful, skilful unpicking of meaning ... is very important.

Conclusion

LAC is an approach to managing the individual children and young people who need out-of-home care in such a way as to ensure maximum possible transparency and accountability as well as inclusion of the child/ young person and their carers in the process of such management. It integrates systematic process with an integrated information system that can inform government policy making if government seeks to use it. It has been Barnardos Australia that has been the lead agency in getting some of the Australian State governments to adopt the LAC approach. Jude Morwitzer in reflecting on this chapter from the vantage point of 2007 (thus four years after we originally interviewed her) comments: 'Further down the track now it is even more apparent that LAC helps to address issues that previously undermined the efficient delivery of service'. The success and sustainability of the LAC approach will depend on the commitment of government at both State and national levels in Australia to provide both direction and resources for an effective and inclusive child and young-person-centred system of out-of-home care.

Notes

1 Steyaert (1997, 13) says of the United Kingdom that the LAC system 'allows the statistical information needs of managers and policy makers to be embedded into an information system that addresses the information needs of the service provider. In that way, it is an integrated information system.' In this section of his article, he says also 'probably because of the high involvement of the state in social service provision in the UK and the scale of social service departments, there is a much higher involvement of computer systems for administrative support in the UK than in other European countries'.

2 At the time of fieldwork, the senior manager (Deidre Dixon) was responsible for the overall coordination and development of The LAC Project and the sale of Australian adapted LAC materials and training to Australian agencies under a commercial license arrangement with the UK Department of Health. She also managed one of Barnardos Australia's seven welfare centres in Sydney. The Program Manager of The LAC Project (Jude Morwitzer) worked on the development of new products to assist agencies in implementation of the LAC system, coordinates LAC training, and works closely with agencies prior to and during LAC implementation (Dixon and Morwitzer 2001).

3 'Towards the end of 2000 ACT became the first Australian State or Territory to initiate full cross-sector (government and non-government agency) implementation for all children in out-of-home care, regardless of auspice agency. This was done as part of a major review of the out-of-home care system in ACT, and contracting out of all care placement services to the nongovernment sector' (Dixon and Morwitzer 2001, 3).

4 It is suggestive on this point that Jude Morwitzer said that new workers embrace LAC more easily than experienced workers. It may not be just that the latter have to adopt a new *modus operandi* when they are comfortable with and experienced in an old one, but that LAC represents more contemporary service norms. We did not probe this point.

10
Care for the Self: 'Community Aged Care Packages'

Michael D. Fine with Anna Yeatman

> ... they've been sending someone in to look after me ever since. I had Ken for a hell of a long while. One of the nicest blokes you'd ever find. When he resigned I had different women ... I got one nice little woman now. A girl. Little Georgie. She's a nice little thing—she runs me everywhere I want to go. In the car. ... Oh she's more of a friend than a carer. ... If I got something to ask them I explain to them they'll sit down and listen. Georgie and I'll sit down and have a cup of coffee together and a bit of a talk and have a smoke together. (Ronnie S, Help at Home Client, formerly homeless and alcoholic, now in social housing with support from a Community Aged Care Package)

Introduction

The demographic pressure of population ageing and the economics of welfare state restructuring have been accompanied by innovation and service redesign across the field of aged care. Central to this process has been the development of community, or better said, home based forms of support, and the introduction of case management practices. These developments have intersected with, and been supported by, the drive towards an increasing recognition of the intended beneficiaries of the care as individuals. Yet, despite the repeated emphasis in policy and much of the literature on building services around the individual, rather than requiring individuals to fit into the service (Davies 1994; Fox and Raphael 1997; Scharf and Wenger 1995), there have been few, if any, attempts to closely examine the meaning of individualized service delivery in the field of aged care.

Individualization is at once a major development in the way that provision of aged care services is conceptualized and provided, and a powerful perspective through which to understand the reconfiguration of aged care in recent decades (Fine 2005b). In this chapter, I use a case study approach to examine the meaning of individualization in an innovative service, the Benevolent Society's *Help at Home* service and to consider the way that principles of individualization have informed the development of policy in the aged care field. The focus in the case study is on the different constructions of the concept of individualization at different levels of the service delivery process. At the macro level of strategic policy, service planning and funding; at the micro level involving the direct interpersonal relationships involved in service delivery to the individual; and at the meso or organizational level, in which organizational resources and staff are marshalled, organized and deployed. The service provider can be seen as an intermediary that translates national policy and priorities into the direct, intimate relationship of care and daily contact with the intended beneficiaries of the program, older people and, where relevant, their families. The recognition of service users as individuals rather than as just members of the policy category of older people who need assistance with the requirements of daily living in the agency's procedure and operational practice is critical to enabling the policy emphasis on individualization to become real at the point of service delivery.

The question of the subject of individualized service delivery also has a particular salience in the field of aged care. With younger people, as would be true of the service users of the disability employment service discussed in Chapter 12, individualized service provision can be understood as a capability building process, thereby helping to shape a mature moral agent capable of exercising a significant degree of autonomy in their dealings with the world. With frail older people these assumptions cannot be made. Here services are oriented to maintaining the capabilities for autonomy of the person and, as necessary, to providing assistance that complements or extends failing capabilities. Service delivery in this field entails profound physical and personal dependency on the part of older people, and if such dependency is to be met in such a way as to accept the older person as an autonomous individual, then there is a complex playing out of relations of power (Kittay 1999 and 2001; Fine 2005a). Attempting to achieve a just and appropriate balance between recognition of the service user as an individual, whose erstwhile capacity for independent action has been compromised by the frailties of old age, and respect for the needs and limits of carers, both formal care staff and informal or family care-givers, poses fundamental dilemmas.

The case study presented here identifies strengths and positive out-comes associated with an individualized approach to aged care. Commencing with an account of the transformation of aged care policy in Australia from a policy based almost exclusively on institutional models of aged care towards a more comprehensive approach centred on a preference for community care, the chapter then outlines the broad direction of reforms in aged care policy in Australia since the 1980s. Following this, we review the conceptualization and development of the Community Aged Care Package (CACP) program by the relevant Commonwealth Government policy department, focusing on the formal policy objectives and the central place given to the recognition of individuals within the emerging policies. The third section of the chapter builds on this account by examining how the CACP policy framework has shaped the service delivery practices of care managers and care workers in the Help at Home program that serves socially disadvantaged older people in need of ongoing care and personal assistance in South-West Sydney.

Home-based care for individuals

From the introduction of specialized aged care services in the 1950s and 1960s until the commencement of wide-scale reforms under the Labor government in the mid-1980s, nursing homes and other residential aged care services dominated long-term care provisions for older people in Australia (Sax 1985; Fine and Stevens 1998; Fine 1999). This pattern of institutional dominance came to be identified as problematic in a series of official public enquiries undertaken in the early 1980s (McLeay 1982; Australian Senate 1985; DCS 1986). In its place came a new emphasis on community care. There were two major rationales advanced for the change. First, an economic rationale concerned the high cost and limited population coverage achieved by relying on institutional provisions. The demographic transformation associated with population ageing, already clearly evident, was forecast to accelerate in the twenty-first century with the consequence that policy makers were eager to find more cost-efficient forms of care to provide for the steadily increasing numbers of older people projected for the twenty-first century. Second, 'frail aged and younger people with disabilities had become better organised and increasingly articulate about their care needs and preferences' (Home and Community Care Review Working Group 1988, 1)[1], and their views influenced the ethos of Commonwealth

Government conceptions of policy and programs in the area of aged and community care. The policy of promoting access to residential care without alternatives was unpopular and did not provide older people or their families with choice. A series of public scandals had raised awareness of nursing home standards and the processes in place for regulating the quality of care (SWAG 1982; McLeay 1982; Australian Senate 1985), adding weight to calls for an alternative form of provision to be made more widely available. The combination of fiscal conservatism and user group pressure supported a shift from institutional care towards a wider range of services that would provide recipients with choice in where they live as well as opportunities to maintain or develop control over their own lives. In addition, within this policy framework, efforts to both humanize and individualized congregate care was also undertaken by the Commonwealth Government.

Historically, institutional or congregate care was associated with a mass management program where inmates were forced to conform with a regime that deprived them of individual identity, as the work of a range of scholarly and other critics made clear in research that began to be influential from the 1960s (Jones and Fowles 1984). These concerns were given voice in Goffman's classic critique of 'total institutions' (Goffman 1968; Jones and Fowles 1984). Those admitted to such an institution, Goffman argued, are required to carry out their daily activity in the immediate company of a large batch of others, where they are 'treated alike and required to do the same thing together' as they are managed according to a single plan imposed from above, which denies opportunities for any inmate to express an individual identity. The result was the 'mortification of the self' (Goffman 1968, 11ff). Each person is thus forced to abandon their sense of individual dignity and personhood, learning that to survive they must forgo their sense of self-worth and autonomous initiative. Instead, adaptation to institutional life requires that they conform to impersonal institutionalized rules and procedures.

The policy process referred to as 'deinstitutionalization' set out to counter this by closing large scale facilities down, as occurred in the field of mental health, and by providing alternative forms of provision, as occurred in aged care (AIHW 2001). The introduction by the Labor government in 1985 of what came to be known as the Aged Care Reform Strategy emphasized the importance of providing potential service users with 'choice' (DCS 1986; DHHCS 1991; Howe 1997). The strategy had economic appeal to government for it sought to finance an expansion of aged care services within an already projected budget for the existing system of residential care facilities. But the broader appeal of the strategy lay in the expansion of community care as an alternative to residential care, and seen to be a more user-responsive system of care. Where institutional care was necessary or maybe preferred, the more individualized model of providing service to people in their own homes could establish a normative framework of expectations for how institutional care might be offered. Non-institutional or community care held the promise of enabling recipients of support to remain in their own homes, maintaining their possessions and setting their own daily routines.

Within a few years of the introduction of the strategy, further development of the philosophy of supporting individuals took place. This involved the principle of planning services around individuals—not planning the needs of individuals around those of services, the introduction of individualized care plans and the use of case management (Ozanne 1990). A strategy for users' rights to lift the quality of care in nursing homes also extended the logic of the individualization of aged care. The title of a major report on the rights of residents in nursing homes and hostels, *'I'm Still an Individual'* (Ronalds 1989), gives an indication of the emphasis placed on the preservation of individuality. Key elements of the approach subsequently adopted included the introduction of legal safeguards such as a charter of residents' rights, the formal recognition of complaints and appeals procedures, and the creation of community visitors positions intended to sustain informal public scrutiny of the operation of these care homes.

Supporting individuals, managing the budget

The individualization of the delivery of welfare services implies the tailoring of the service to fit the preferences and circumstances of the individual recipient, along with the provision of opportunities for the recipient to take part in the decision making concerned with the planning, organization and delivery of the particular service concerned. The transformation of care services is indicative of a wider process of social change, through which people are increasingly called upon to exercise their own agency, as autonomous adult beings, rather than relying on decision making by others. Yet, in contrast to reforms introduced in many other areas of welfare in which the emphasis is placed on requiring potential beneficiaries to assume responsibility for their own well-being, those introduced into aged care tacitly acknowledge the life course-related dependency of old age. Their focus is not on capability building for service users, but on the recognition of the individuality and remaining capabilities of those who are dependent. This involves an attempt to provide the service recipient with opportunities to sustain a sense of personal dignity through exercising choice. Rather than by forcing them to fit into an expensive but highly ordered system of institutional support and accommodation, individualization is also achieved through the more cost-effective process of building community-based services around their needs.

The approach adopted is also suggestive of a rethinking of what can be termed the 'carer-dependent paradigm' (Fine and Glendinning 2005). In place of the hierarchical pattern of the assumption of responsibility and control by the caregiver or care staff and the expression of passivity and gratitude by the care recipient, a role pattern theorized by Talcott Parsons as 'the sick role' in the 1950s (Parsons 1951; 1957), a more engaged, active, decision making relationship came to be expected. The recipient of care, in this more contemporary approach, is expected to become an active rather than passive agent in the care relationship. The emphasis on individual capacities which are already present and need to be respected and fostered (Wilson 1994), and the concept of the 'least restrictive alternative' (Wolfensberger 1972; Burchard and Clarke 1990) encountered in the field of disability services, capture in many ways the sense in which individuals were acknowledged in the aged care reforms outlined above. Care, in this sense, came to be seen in policy not simply as a one-directional service undertaken by the staff, but as the outcome of a negotiated relationship between the different parties in which the fostering of the service user's capabilities and autonomy is foremost.

Individualized care packages

Community Aged Care Packages (CACPs) were introduced in Australia in 1992, to provide an alternative to low-level residential care[2] for older people in need of ongoing care and support. Their forerunner was the hostel options project in 1991, which allowed hostels to deliver personal care services to persons living at home up to a maximum cost equivalent to the Personal Care Subsidy (Gibson 1998, 38). This was a policy initiative from senior policy makers of the (then) Department of Health and Community Services to deal with a shortage of aged care hostel accommodation which was not being developed at a sufficiently rapid rate to meet the levels of provision required under the Australian government's 'benchmark' for residential care (Mathur, Evans and Gibson 1997; Gibson 1998). At the time, this provided for 100 residential care beds for every 1,000 people aged 70 years or over-40 of these were to be nursing home beds, of which there was a surplus, 60 were to be hostel beds, of which there was a marked shortage. Initiatives to encourage the development of new hostel accommodation had failed, opening the way for the proposal of a new form of provision that could help the Labor government of the time achieve the desired level of provision: 'packages' of aged care were to be provided to older people formally assessed by an Aged Care Assessment Team (ACATs) as needing ongoing residential care, but unable to obtain it in their local area.[3] The packages of care were an innovative approach to service delivery that separated the residential aspect of hostel service from the care and support services provided in the facility. Instead of bundling care and accommodation together as a single service, CACPs were intended to enable the same level of care and support to be provided to those assessed as eligible for residential care but who remained in their own home. CACPs thus originated not as a grass roots initiative in service delivery, but as a centralized policy measure introduced at the most senior levels of the public service.

The program has been expanded consistently since its introduction in 1992. By 1996 there were 4,196 packages provided by 242 approved services in Australia, a rate of approximately 2.9 packages per thousand people aged 70 years and over (Mathur, Evans and Gibson 1997). Their number has since increased considerably. As CACPs gained acceptance from both consumers and the Commonwealth government their part in the residential care 'benchmark' increased, with the goal going from 0 in 1992 to ten packages per thousand aged 70 or over by 1995 (DHSH 1995), and 15 places/1,000 in early 2002 (see Table 10.1). The current 'planning framework' aims to provide 88 residential aged care places (covering high

Table 10.1   Number of operational Community Aged Care Packages and the provision ratio per 1,000 persons aged 70 years and over, 1992 to 2005

Year	Community Aged Care Packages	Packages per 1,000 Persons Aged 70 years and Over[a]
1992	235	0.2
1996	4,431	2.9
2000	18,309	10.8
2004	29,063	15.6
2005	30,916	17.2

Source: Australian Institute of Health and Welfare (AIHW) 2003a. *Community Aged Care Packages in Australia 2001–02: a statistical overview*. AIHW cat. no. AGE 30. Canberra: AIHW (Aged Care Statistics Series no. 14): 2; AIHW 2005: *Australia's Welfare 2005*: 191; AIHW 2007 *Aged Care Packages in the Community* 2005–06, viii.
(a) The ratios are those pertaining on 30 June each year. They are based on ABS population estimates and are recalculated back to 1997. From 2000, the data in this table include packages provided by Multi-Purpose Services and flexible funding under the Aboriginal and Torres Strait Islander Aged Care Strategy.

and low care places) and 20 places in the community (mainly CACPs), for every 1,000 people aged 70 years and over (plus Aboriginal and Torres Strait Islander people aged between 50 and 69 years) (CACP Guidelines 2004: Section 7).

The Program Guidelines for CACPs identify eligible recipients as

> frail older people (generally considered to be aged 70 and older for non-Indigenous people, and 50 years and over for Indigenous people) living in the community *who would be assessed by an Aged Care Assessment Team as eligible to receive at least low level residential aged care, if they applied,* and who have,

> a. complex care needs arising from physical, social and psychological needs;
> b. a need for a coordinated package of care services;
> c. a preference to remain living in the community with appropriate and reliable supports;
> d. a need for ongoing monitoring and review of changing care needs; and
> e. the ability to live in the community with appropriate community care (CACP Guidelines 2004: Section 2.2, emphasis in original).[4]

The phrase 'complex care needs' covers the pattern of multiple medical conditions and functional impairment that typically characterize the profile of frailty in old age. It indicates the complex interconnections between somatic, emotional, psychological and social dimensions of such frailty. Many older applicants for assistance experience a compounded effect of frailty on some or all of these dimensions, and they need assistance with a variety of the activities of daily living (ADLs) as well as with other more episodic activities such as attending medical appointments.

While assessment for eligibility focuses on individual applicants, there is also recognition given to the socio-economic-cultural position of applicants. Under the *Aged Care Act 1997* (Section 12–15), priority of access is to be given to 'special needs groups', which include people who are from non-English speaking backgrounds; from Aboriginal and Torres Strait Islander communities; who live in rural or remote areas; or who are financially or socially disadvantaged (CACP Guidelines 1999: 6).

Despite the increasing significance of CACPs for aged care in Australia, there are few published studies. Information publicly available is at the level of data analyses and policy indicators, concerning such issues as the aggregate levels of provision and comparative client dependency.

When CACP clients are compared with the recipients of hostel level care (Mathur, Evans and Gibson 1997; Gibson and Mathur 1999) for example, it has been found there while there is some overlap in the client groups served, there are also some distinct differences, suggesting that despite the origins of aged care packages as a substitute for low-level residential care, the programs are not full equivalents as the CACP population, by and large, is somewhat less disabled and more independent.

Packaging services for individuals

Care packages provide the opportunity for providers to adjust service to match the needs of individual recipients. Program guidelines emphasize the link to individual consumers.

> A key feature of the CACP Program is the provision of individually tailored packages of care services that are planned and managed by an Approved Provider. The program requires all older people to be assessed by an Aged Care Assessment Team (ACAT). The services provided as part of a CACP are designed to meet people's daily care needs and may vary as an individual's care needs change. (CACP Guidelines 2004: Section 1)

The guidelines continue,

> CACPs are individually planned and coordinated packages of community aged care services, designed to meet older people's daily care needs in the community. CACPs are targeted at frail older people living in the community who require management of services because of their complex care needs. These people would otherwise be eligible for at least low level residential care. (CACP Guidelines 2004: Section 2)

The emphasis on tailoring services to the individual has to be reconciled with other responsibilities of the service provider to integrate the service with the wider service system, to respect staff rights, and to comply with other policy and administrative requirements. A number of conditions are outlined that are central to the understanding of the notion of individualized service delivery fostered in the program. This requires that the approved service provider should:

a. have a commitment to the provision of an individual package of services, tailored to the needs of care recipients, who are active participants in planning their own care;

b. provide a structure which creates or facilitates integration with any existing service system and the community assisted by the service;
c. put in place administrative arrangements, policies and procedures which support and protect the rights of staff; and
d. ensure accountability while encouraging an innovative approach to service provision. (CACP Guidelines 2004: Section 6)

The first of these conditions suggests that the package of services needs not only to be 'tailored' to the individual, but that the process requires the active participation of the recipient in planning the care to be provided. Given the prevalence of dementia amongst potential applicants, a level of 'active participation' may at times be difficult to attain. However, it provides a normative indicator of what is to be striven for—providers are not to be in a position of imposing preconceived service measures on the recipient.

In the context of caring for older people in their own home, concern for the fostering of links with other services (as set out in point b. above), for the well-being of staff and for accountability procedures for service providers is not merely a matter of risk management. The issue of the 'integration' of service provision picks up on recognition of this issue in the field of service delivery for older people and on evidence that reliance on a number of highly specialized services can be an alienating and fragmenting experience for consumers (Fine 1998). Identifying the issues of the need to support and protect staff, and the importance of accountability of the service managers (point c. above) also points to important constraints on the 'individualization' of service delivery. Care is a social relationship in which the rights and obligations of each party must be recognized. What counts as individualization from the service user's perspective has to be reconcilable with the rights of service workers.

Care packages rely on the use of a case management approach to provide an integrated package of assistance that tailors the mix of personal and care services to the needs of individual recipients. How this is done depends very much on the provider agency. It is possible to link recipients into the system of services provided by residential facilities, but most providers rely on a specialized workforce. The program guidelines point out that providers 'should not be constrained by standard patterns or practices of service delivery but can develop creative responses which may include the contracting of private individuals or agencies' (CACP Guidelines 1999: 17).

Public responsibility and individualized funding mechanisms

CACPs are funded directly by the Australian Government with a pre-scribed and nationally standardized level of user contributions. The basis of funding is by daily subsidy paid to providers for approved care recipients occupying approved care package places. The subsidy rate in September 2003 was AUD 11,465 per person per annum or AUD 31.41 per client per day. Users of care packages are required to pay a fee to contribute to the cost of their package up to a maximum of 17.5% of the basic rate of single pension. For the majority of users dependent on the Aged Pension this contribution was AUD 5.45 per day in 2003. There is provision for users with additional income over the basic pension where providers may charge up to an additional 50% of the income above the basic pension.

The funding level for CACPs effectively prescribes in broad terms the actual levels of paid assistance it is possible to provide CACP recipients. In 2002, the median numbers of hours help received by users across Australia was 5.5 hours per week, the average 6.1 hours (AIHW 2003a, 64). These figures work out at slightly less than an hour per day. The average, however, disguises considerable variation in the hours of assist-ance provided. Almost one in ten users (9.6%) received ten hours of help or more in the same week. Although no maximum number of hours is set, the financial limits effectively mean that there is an absolute limit of around 14 hours per week. To achieve this, a local provider would need to internally redistribute resources between users, ensuring that other users within the scheme received below the average hours.

In this way, the program of community care packages sets a strong financial upper limit on the amount of assistance that can be provided to an individual recipient, just as the assessment and eligibility require-ments, set out in the program guidelines, determine a fairly strict entry threshold. The high floor and low ceiling of the program (Howe 1994), effectively contain the scope of CACPs by constraining their capacity to provide ongoing care to the individuals who rely on the assistance they provide to keep them in their own home. If a recipient's needs for support increase it may be possible to keep them in the program for a short time, but it is not possible to continue service for a prolonged period. Instead, if they wish to continue to receive support they must transfer to another program. Consequently, many of those on a care package only receive it for a short time before they either move on to the more intensive forms of support provided in residential care, or die.

In the most recent national census of the program, 27% had received help for less than six months, while 63%, almost two in every three recipients of assistance, had been on the program for less than 18 months.

The public funding model has strong individualized payment elements based on a direct match between an individual user and the funded place s/he receives. Funding is tied to individual packages of care in a manner directly comparable to the funding of residential care beds, effectively guaranteeing each service user a secure level of service resources. Furthermore, the funding system effectively safeguards each package. Contrast this with the block funding system used for services funded through the Home and Community Care (HACC) program, where funding is paid directly to the service concerned but is not linked to a fixed number of places. Faced with evidence of heightened demand, HACC providers can use the flexibility of the program's funding provisions to stretch their service capacity, assisting additional clients by reducing the average hours of service each client receives, spreading service more thinly. The rationing system inherent in linking a fixed number of CACP places to a fixed number of individual users, in contrast, means that when demand exceeds existing capacity, waiting lists grow. At local level these can often be six to 12 months long, or longer. This means that it is often difficult and sometimes impossible for an approved applicant to gain a place, even after a full assessment has been made by an Aged Care Assessment Team (ACAT) and eligibility determined beyond doubt.

One of the key changes made to the operation of CACPs by the Coalition government 1996 has been to open up their provision to for-profit providers. However there is no evidence of significant expansion of corporate interest in the field to date, and the program continues to be predominantly one operated by non-profit agencies, with over 95% of the 759 outlets included in the most recently available census defining themselves as 'not for profit' (AIHW 2004: 27, 73).[5]

Help at home[6]

The Benevolent Society, founded in 1820 with help from Governor Macquarie, then governor of the newly established colony of New South Wales, is claimed to be Australia's oldest non-government provider of welfare and support services (Dickey 1980). Its provision of services is now directed to three major client groups: older people; women; and children in care. Until the mid-1990s the Benevolent Society's aged care services were exclusively residential care facilities—nursing homes and hostels. Since then there has been a deliberate effort to expand services delivered to people who remain in their own homes. This has been achieved mainly through competing for funding from the Australian government for additional CACP places, although there are now also some other services in some areas of Sydney funded through the Home and Community Care (HACC) program. This study focuses on just one project, the *Help at Home* service, based in Bexley and operating in neighbouring areas of Southern Sydney.

Currently, the Benevolent Society is funded to provide 96 CACP places in the Southern Sydney area, spread over two projects that together form the Help at Home service: 34 of these are in the Riverwood project, 62 in the Canterbury area. The Help at Home project, particularly the Riverwood service which is based on a large Housing Department public housing complex, represents an explicit commitment from the Benevolent Society to support disadvantaged older people to gain or maintain control over their life circumstances and remain in their own home, despite significant levels of disability, social isolation and, in many instances, life-long experiences of social and economic adversity. Many of the Help at Home clients have been assisted to become tenants in Housing Commission and other social housing accommodation by the Benevolent Society. Others remain in their own homes. A total of 34 funded places are 'housing linked packages' developed specifically to enable those with severe social disadvantage, typically with a background of homelessness, alcoholism, mental illness or a history of imprisonment. These clients are often socially isolated and incapable of continuing to live on their own without assistance. Some, for example, were convicted criminals with histories of imprisonment. Many others had been homeless. A brief statistical overview of the Help at Home clients in March 2003 is presented in Table 10.2.

Funding for the Riverwood project, in 2003, involved an annual government subsidy of AUD 381,000 and client fees of AUD 15,000. This covered the wages and other costs of one full-time Coordinator (responsible for case management) and eight part-time care workers, as well as part of the other administrative and organizational costs incurred.

Operation of the Help at Home service

Help at Home operates in the socially deprived suburb of Riverwood and in the Canterbury area of Sydney, providing case managed assistance to older people who remain in their own home or who

Table 10.2   Clients assisted by the Help at Home Program, 2003

	Riverwood		Canterbury	
	Male	Female	Male	Female
Clients (n)	15	19	20	42
Marital status				
Single	5	2	3	2
Divorced/widowed	7	16	7	32
Married/partner	3	1	10	8
Age (years)				
Less than 60	0	1	0	1
61–70	0	1	2	0
71–80	6	6	5	7
81–90	7	9	10	23
91–100	2	2	2	11
Dwelling				
Own home	5	6	19	39
Private rental	4	3	1	2
Public rental	6	10	0	1
House	6	8	18	31
Flat	9	11	2	11
Income				
Pension only	10	18	12	31
Pension + own	3	1	5	1
Own income	2	0	2	2
Length of service				
Less than 6 month	6	7	0	2
6–12 months	1	2	12	14
1–2 years	4	2	4	9
2–3 years	1	2	3	5
3–4 years	0	1	0	11
4 years +	3	5	1	1

have been placed in social housing owned by the New South Wales Department of Housing, or rented privately. To be eligible to receive assistance, all clients must first be assessed by one of the regional Aged Care Assessment Teams as requiring a level of support equal to that of the low-level residential care. Often a period of waiting is required following that assessment until a CACP place becomes vacant. Following that, a service assessment is made by a care coordinator (case manager) from Help at Home. Typically, this involves the Coordinator matching the new client to a care worker, introducing the care worker to the client with the service proceeding. In many cases getting the client to accept the service requires careful and patient negotiation. One such case involved a client assessed by the ACAT at Canterbury as being capable of remaining in her own home, but needing much more help, particularly in the form of ongoing personal support, than she currently received.

One of the two full-time Help at Home care coordinators with whom I worked, Vicky, came to collect me to accompany her on her first visit to Mrs D. in her home in a nearby suburb. Mrs D. doesn't want help from Help at Home, she said, but without it is likely to be placed in a home. Vicky's plan is to become familiar and trusted and work herself slowly into a position where she could provide help.[7]

The home is a large double fronted brick house that looks like it has seen better days. We rang the door bell several times but there was initially no answer. Finally, after a phone call it was opened a little, and a small frail older woman in her late 80s appeared. Her hands were contorted with arthritis. Wearing a cotton night dress, she was otherwise friendly and seemed intelligent. She complained about the neighbours parking in front of her house and about her brother and his son, who, she told us, could not be trusted anymore. She said she had asked her younger brother to help her if ever she needed it, and trusted him. Now he wanted her out of the house, she said. The conversation went on, as she explained how she had survived a cancer operation on her bowels. She would understand it if, when she returned to the doctor, he told her it had come back. She'd book herself into a hospice for the dying, she said, but till then she was going to stay in the house and didn't need help, thank you. The community nurse who came most days was very help-ful and she also had help from the Home Care service who were often good, although she didn't trust them after something was 'stolen'. ...

She told us she accepts help and advice from the home nurse, so Vicky resolved to call her and to send a Care Worker to accompany the nurse next week, if possible. Vicky told me she didn't want to have to go to the Guardianship Board over this, as that would break Mrs D's heart and drain her will to live. Far better to work slowly to gain her trust. That's one of the most satisfying feelings when it works, Vicky told me.

Developing trust between clients, care workers and coordinators is one of the keys to the Help at Home approach. The personal relationship between case managers, other care staff and clients helps enable clients to feel that they are not being subjected to an imposed formal and official intervention. They are not 'treated like a number' as one client described it, but more like a friend or family member. Many of the service's clients, indeed, had a life history filled with hostile or humiliating encounters with the authorities, and were reluctant to allow another impersonal agency to take control once again.

Each care coordinator was responsible for the care of up to 40 clients. Their task is to get to know the client and establish a relationship of trust and respect while making a detailed assessment of the work of care and support required. This builds on the formal medical/social assessment undertaken at the referral stage by the ACAT, but needs to be quite practical in working out the day-to-day support arrangements that will be viable over the longer term. These are often tentatively worked out into a weekly program. Once this is achieved, each client is assigned a carefully matched care worker who in turn works to build a personal relationship with the client while undertaking the support tasks required. Unlike staff of most specialized community care services, the care worker is multi-tasked and responsible for a very broad range of activities, from personal care to housecleaning, cooking and assistance with shopping, financial management and medical appointments. The care worker is thus assigned considerable responsibility for providing ongoing assistance to the client, and is supported by the coordinator/case manager in dealing with the practical issues and emotional support that was required.

The aspect of people work, of enabling the care worker to find meaning in her or his work through building a personal relationship with the client, was important for care workers as well as clients. For example, Michelle, an Australian born mother of four who worked part-time as a care worker, spoke about her work as involving personally fulfilling relationships that help clients realize their own goals, in particular that of remaining at home.

(Why do I like it?) Just to see that they're happy. To know that they're with their family, they're in their own environment which they've always been in, not to be put into a nursing home that's a poky little room that has everything in the one room. Toilet, laundry, whatever, all in the same room—I just don't think that's right—they don't deserve it. They're the ones that brought us up and now we're looking after them. ... They become friends. Even though your boss tells you, and they do, 'please don't get attached, don't get too involved', you can't help but get involved with them because they're lovely people and it's just something that you're giving them back what they gave to you. Maybe not exactly them, but it's my way of saying thank you to my mum and dad. I will be able to do that for my mum and dad when they get to that age, but at present that's how I do it. I quite enjoy it. ... You do get involved, you can't help it. It's like being a nurse. You do get attached. So you do have to learn to pull away, but you work with it and you just work through it. Like anything, if you're strong you can do it, if you're not, look out.

The success of the relationships established between care workers and clients can be traced back to the foundations established by the care coordinators and, in turn, shaped by the program guidelines. Vicky, the care coordinator referred to by Michelle as her 'boss', described it as follows:

As coordinators I guess our role is to start from the very beginning with the client so although we receive assessments from ACAT, we also do our own assessments and ensure the client is able to come on to our package at the level of care that meets their needs. So we do the assessment, then we do the care plan. So we build a care plan with the client and then we go on then to place a care worker with that client. The care plan is individual—it's different for every client. And then I guess it's just case managing that ... the issues can be so varied and as case managers a lot of our time is also spent on rostering and supervising care workers, so we manage between 16–20 care workers. Each coordinator has that team. There's that aspect as well.

... I think also we can provide a good service because the care workers are actually very committed to what they do. They see the same people every day. In nursing homes often they're there for a shift and they're pushed for time and everything's rushed and although our care workers are rushed there's no question about it, they have a real commitment to this person and often will see them through really difficult times. The client can trust the care worker and they often become a part of their lives. That's really important and it actually adds another dimension to their lives. I think that's something we can do with packages as well, that isn't so possible in institutions.

The process of helping care workers develop such a relationship with clients takes time and effort, assessing clients, and matching staff in order to create the conditions for trust.

So I'll often put off having a client start on the service, for example this client now that I won't put on until somebody gets back from leave, because I think she's the right person for this client. We had a situation earlier this year where I had a client who waited for seven weeks because I knew that if we didn't have the right care worker it wasn't going to work. It's worked beautifully, so you're better off taking your time in the initial process, making sure that client's supported obviously and then it'll work. I think it's the most important part of the process.

Measures were also developed to monitor client's behaviour and to intervene where problems developed. This was particularly important where dementia might be involved.

Recognition of the individual's sense of self is, thus, central to the Help at Home's approach to service delivery. At the point at which the service or its agents directly interact with service users, recognition of the individual is conceived operationally as actions that commence with listening to the individual service user to determine what it is s/he wants to achieve, then working to enable the person to achieve these goals. Typically, this involves helping them to remain in their own home. If service users want to stay at home, it was considered the duty of the Help at Home service to help them realize that goal as far as was considered congruent with their welfare. But there is also an open acknowledgement of the need to assume responsibility for the individual's well being, including, if necessary, maintaining control of certain everyday decisions. For example, in one instance I observed it was necessary to stop a client from hoarding food. This was achieved by delivering or preparing three small meals each day, so that there would be no leftovers. Keeping a vigilant eye on her to keep her safe was made central to the care plan as a measure that was necessary to enable her to attain her own goal of remaining safely in her own home for as long as possible. Thus as with the community care practice in the United Kingdom researched by Chris Clark (1998), a professional paternalism co-exists with and sometimes overrides respect for the self-determination of the service user. As Clark (1998, 389) suggests, the rationale for and limits of paternalism—meaning inter-vention 'on the grounds of someone's interests without his or her fully informed consent'—in community care is neglected in contemporary conceptions of person-centred care even though practitioners are fully aware of having to juggle paternalistic considerations and respect for the person's wishes:

> Social workers [in community care practice] clearly grasp that sometimes self-determination must give way to over-riding considerations for the client's safety and welfare in the face of serious risk. Paternalistic intervention—in the shape of overpower-ing influence and persuasion (often by the offer or withholding of resources), legal compulsion, deliberate deception or the withhold-ing of information—is accepted with reluctance, as occasionally necessary. The pivotal question in deciding whether paternalism is justified is the determination of mental competence ... (Clark 1998, 397).

For both clients and staff, an important feature that enables the service to acknowledge the client as an individual is the opportunity to get to know him or her over a prolonged period. This is as impor-tant for the building of trust, through which the client can learn to rely on the care staff, as it is the building of familiarity between staff and client. Here it is important to distinguish between respect-ing the individual's wishes in the sense of allowing them to be the determining arbiter of action taken, and developing a service response that is oriented to the way of being in the world that is this indi-vidual's, and, so far as possible, respecting his or her wishes. If the service actually meets the concrete specificity of this individual's way of being, then staff are doing their level best to honour and secure this individual's sense of self. For this to be possible, staff have to be able to get to know the individual and vice versa. Michael, the other care coordinator with whom I worked closely, described it as follows:

> One of the main differences in this job is that you can potentially develop a relationship with a client that extends over a long period of time and that in itself can have a really big impact on the kind of

service they receive. Because the more you get to know them, the more they trust you, the easier it is to navigate around somebody who might have a dementia who might otherwise be distrustful of services coming in. If you can get to know them over a period of time there's a lot more depth to what you can actually do with someone.

For case managers and care workers, recognizing the client as an individual was inconceivable without acknowledging the person's life history and their continuing links with others, including family members, neighbours and friends. Developing relationships with their families and the neighbours was therefore regarded as essential.

Conclusion

Today, most services in the field of aged care endeavour to offer greater recognition to the client as an individual than in the past. This has been achieved through the re-structuring of service organization along such lines as patient or person-centred care, through the use of case or care management and the introduction of a variety of personalized programs in evidence (Clark 1998; Feinberg and Ellano 2000; Glendinning *et al.* 2000; Fisher and Fine 2002). In many instances, these have been accompanied by moves for improved legal protection of consumers through advocacy and user rights provisions. The extent to which these goals move beyond rhetoric and policy to be realized in practice, however, remains a challenge to service providers and policy makers.

In the case of Community Aged Care Packages we have an innovative program in which the principles of individualized service delivery have been made a central design feature. Noteworthy is the degree of integration of this design feature at all levels of the service system concerned: the policy, program management and service agency levels. This is a case where policy oriented to population management (the 'ageing of society') is also oriented to the principle of individualization and where, accordingly, there is a top-down strategy for a systemic integration of principles of tight fiscal management, demographically-based health and welfare planning and individualization in aged care. This strategy has been evolving in Australia since the mid-1980s, and it has created a relatively stable environment for service provision and service user expectations.

In the case of the Community Aged Care Packages, a specific component of the Australian aged care system, they have been increasing consistently since their introduction in 1992. Unlike other welfare sectors, then, where unmet need has either remained constant or grown over the period of time that the rhetoric of individualization (person-centred care) has been adopted by government as the funding agency, this is a sector where service growth has been ambitiously attempting to expand to match the growth of need. In this context, service agencies responsible for the provision of CACPs can plan for service growth and development in a context where they are free to accumulate learning from their experience of how to individualize service delivery.

Notes

1 The synergy across self advocates in both groups —frail older people and younger people with disabilities—was made possible by the integrated conception of home and community care in both legislation and policy, a conception that translated into program design that lasted until 1990. The integrated conception was expressed in the idea that it was functional disability and the need for assistance in meeting the tasks of everyday living that was the service focus of the HACC program. '*The Home and Community Care Act 1985* subsumed four existing Commonwealth Acts, expanding the client group from primarily aged persons to include younger people with disabilities and informal carers and increasing the range of services eligible for funding. Perhaps most importantly from the users' point of view, the Act removed the legislative barriers between the four former Acts enabling the focus to be changed from providing particular types of service (e.g. home care, delivered meals, home nursing) to providing a coordinated set of services to satisfy individuals' assessed needs (Home and Community Care Review Working Group 1988, 1–2)'.

2 In the Australian system of old aged services, the lower level of residential care is called hostel care, while the more intensive level of care is called nursing home care.

3 In the development of a tightly fiscally and bureaucratically managed system of aged care, Australia developed the ACAT model as only authorized point of assessment for determining whether publicly funded (or subsidized) old aged care was to be allocated, at what level and of what type.

4 Revised, but incomplete, program guidelines were released in November 2004. Where ever possible these, rather than earlier guidelines, have been cited. In some instances details of the sections of the guidelines are not available, with the effect that earlier provisions continue to apply. These have been cited where applicable.

5 This situation is in marked contrast to that evident in other service fields, such as residential aged care and child care in Australia, in which corporate for-profit providers have expanded massively, dominating provision (Fine 1999; AIHW 2003b).

6 The case study was conducted using an ethnographic approach, using participant observation and in-depth interviews over a four-month period, from November 2002 to March 2003. Extensive use has also been made of documentary materials and publications produced by BenSoc. The study is not an

attempt to analyse or evaluate the CACP program as a whole. Nor is it clear to what extent any of the reported findings could be generalized to other sites, agencies or projects. A number of unique features of provision which make it unlikely that the Help at Home project is 'typical' of the way that other community aged care packages are delivered in Australia. Instead, this case study was chosen to provide a compelling exemplar with which to test out the issues involved in translating the injunction to provide an individualized form of service delivery to those who are unlikely to overcome their dependent social or financial status, and for whom no hopes are possible for promoting a move to greater levels of independence.

7 This and other extracts is based on my fieldwork notes and interviews. The names of all clients have been changed to protect confidentiality. Staff members are referred to by their first name as they have indicated was their preference.

11

Service Delivery and HIV-Positive Gay Men: Pre- and Post-Advent of Highly Active Antiretroviral Treatment (HAART)

Anna Yeatman and Gary W. Dowsett

Introduction

The HIV/AIDS pandemic has posed and continues to pose unique challenges for service delivery, and it is the nature of these challenges to require us to think about the idea of service delivery in a more complex way than normally occurs. Medical and pharmaceutical interventions in relation to the virus are not sufficient; or, rather, these types of intervention have to be embedded within education, prevention, and illness management approaches that take account of both the lived experience of individuals and its contextualization within the sociology of the epidemic and the sexual cultures (Dowsett 2006) with which it is entwined.

In this chapter our focus is on service delivery pre and post the advent in 1996 of the new highly active antiretroviral treatment (HAART) for people who are HIV positive with specific reference to gay men in Australia. The prominence of the medical management of the disease is inevitable but its significance changes depending on which of these two periods is in view. Moreover, the medical management of this disease is uniquely situated for several reasons. Firstly, many of the treating doctors have been gay men themselves, some of whom died in the pre-treatments stage of the epidemic. Secondly, this is still a mortal disease but in the post-treatments era people who are positive and using treatments are staying alive for relatively long periods of time compared with the pre-treatments era. This places HIV treatment doctors in a particularly complex relationship of collaborating with their individual patients over a relatively long period of time where the treatments involve difficult issues concerning both side-effects and how they impact on the individual patient's management of their daily life routines. Thirdly, as

Alison Moore (2005, 105) observes, HIV medicine is a 'complex context that involves making decisions about powerful, toxic and (at the time) relatively untested drug regimens, against the backdrop of the highly politicized field of gay community self-determination'. This is an area where the patient constituency has a history of forceful political mobilization, where as already suggested many of the professionals serving this constituency share that history, and where, in addition, there has been a rich and ongoing learning experience on the part of gay-identified activists who have self-selected into managing and containing the epidemic in the gay male community.

In no other area of medicine does there seem to be this confluence of factors that make for an extraordinarily dense and creative point of encounter between medicine and the life worlds as well as lived bodies of those who need medical intervention. Here biomedicine both as clinical and research practice has to work with the 'lived body' of those who need it (for these two terms of corporeality, see Rothfield 1997). Moreover, as Dowsett (2006) suggests, just how HIV-positive status is lived, and attributed meaning, by gay men is itself a set of cultural dynamics that is informed by past historical experience. Dowsett (2006, 16) suggests that contemporary gay sexual cultures are imbued with nuanced and complex responses to earlier prevention education campaigns in ways that need to be understood:

> It is interesting to speculate if diversifying approaches to condom use from the unitary 'safe sex every time' message might have incited potential shifts in sexual safety among gay men, particularly as there has never been full compliance any way. For example, we can never know whether an increased interest in the practice of anal sex is a consequence of the development of modern gay communities, or of the emphasis we have placed upon that practice over the last twenty plus years in HIV prevention. After all, and as one example, nearly 90% of gay men in Sydney now practice it with regular partners and just on 80% with casual partners. There has been a steady reported increase in the practice since 1996, and levels are significantly higher than in the first Australian HIV study in 1986.

The history of the HIV-AIDS epidemic in Australia so far

The first AIDS diagnosis in Australia was in 1982 (Dowsett 2003,123). The Australian HIV epidemic has been primarily an epidemic associated with male-to-male sex.[1] It is for this reason that the gay community has been so prominent in the Australian response to the epidemic and it is also why gay community activism has been the modality of PLWHA (People living with HIV-AIDS) activism in the Australian context. For reasons largely to do with a reform-oriented federal state at the time when the Australian epidemic got under way there has been a remarkably successful strategy for the containment of epidemic undertaken by the Australian State in partnership with the communities most at risk of HIV transmission (the gay community, sex workers, and intravenous drug users). The national AIDS strategy began in 1984 and continues until the present.[2]

The Australian State brokered a stakeholder partnership across public officials in relevant state administrative line agencies, medical researchers, social researchers, and gay community activists that provided the architecture of the policy, research and service response to HIV treatment, prevention and education. The Australian government's response came early in the epidemic; the Medical Working Party on AIDS was established in 1983 under the auspices of the National Health and Medical Research Council, it was re-formed in 1984, and it became the National AIDS taskforce in 1985 (Dowsett 1998, 179; see also Ballard 1998). A parallel National Advisory Committee of AIDS was also established at that time, whose membership included a wide range of non-medical and affected-community voices, and whose tasks *inter alia* were to advise and stimulate prevention programs and community responses in care and support for PLWHA. There are two national peak bodies representing Australians who live with the virus: the Australian Federation of AIDS Organisations (AFAO) which is self-designated as 'the national federation for the HIV community response' that provides 'leadership coordination and support to the national policy, advocacy and health promotion response to HIV/AIDS' (AFAO website downloaded March 31, 2008); and the National Association of People Living with HIV/AIDS (NAPWA) which represents the needs of HIV+ people to government and the pharmaceutical industry, pursues a partnership approach working alongside the policy makers, HIV clinicians, researchers, the pharmaceuticals, consumer health and disability groups, participates in community-based education strategies, and works with service providers to ensure that the needs of HIV+ people are met (NAPWA website downloaded March 31, 2008).

Thus central to the development of service design and service delivery in the response to the epidemic has been a complex field of stakeholders whose combined presence has articulated the distinctive stakes of public health, public policy and administration, the drug companies, medical research, social research, and the social movement representing those most at risk of HIV transmission. For this reason it is impossible to think of service delivery in relation to HIV in the Australian case without reference to this complex mix of political, professional, and, as it is now, professional-activist as well as consumer interests in the effective management of the epidemic.

The pandemic has had two major phases divided by the development of antiviral drugs which help stop HIV from infecting new cells in the individual's body. Combination therapy or the combined use of usually three or four drugs has been the basis of treatment since 1996. While the use of combination HIV therapies known as HAART can have serious side effects that have a negative impact on the quality of life of those who take these drugs, their introduction caused an immediate decline in HIV deaths and brought about the end of the phase of the epidemic that was associated with high mortality and the personal as well as collective trauma it visited on gay men, their individual networks of significant others, and the gay community. The new HIV therapies are not a magic potion: this summary from US-based researchers can be generalized to other contexts in the developed world where the combination therapies have been in use for almost a decade:

> There are recent indications that the rate of decline in HIV deaths and serious illness has slowed ... evidence of resistance to HIV medications among newly infected patients is mounting. Drug resistance compromises an individual's chances for optimal HIV care and long-term quality of life and may eventually pose a widespread public health threat from HIV resistant strains (Noring *et al.* 2001, 693).

The importance of preventing transmission remains as important as it ever was, especially in the face of evidence of a newly increasing rate of HIV transmission in male-to-male sex throughout the first half of this decade (now thought to be leveling off), and thus ongoing attention to services aimed at educating those at risk of HIV transmission in prevention practices continues to be central to the management of the epidemic.

At the same time education and health promotion oriented to reduction of HIV transmission has become more complex in a context where HIV-positive gay men are living with the illness rather than dying—as was the case prior to the introduction of antiviral drugs—and continue to be sexually active. This is also a context where since 1996 new pathology techniques have made the measurement of viral load a clinical tool for determining how much HIV is in the blood of someone who is HIV-positive. Now it is not just a matter of negotiating safe sex in terms of establishing seroconcordance with a known partner (both being positive or negative), but there are more nuanced risk reduction strategies adopted as when, for example, someone who has seroconverted (tested as HIV+ for the first time) has an undetectable viral load and assumes that there is low risk of transmission in unprotected anal intercourse (see for discussion of risk reduction strategies Rosengarten *et al.* 2000). The factors that make contemporary HIV education considerably more difficult and complex for the gay male community at this time also include what various commentators describe as an end to a sense of crisis, complacency, safe sex fatigue, treatment optimism, and the coming onto the scene of younger gay men who have not been acculturated within the gay community's lived experience of the history of the epidemic (see Rosengarten *et al.* 2000; Dowsett 2006).

With the development of the availability of antiretroviral drugs, their impact on slowing the epidemic, and on keeping people living with the virus alive, there has been a dramatic shift in the collective subjectivity that marked the pre- and post-combination therapy eras. At the time of a high rate of mortality the impact of which was felt within a highly compressed period of time, there was a collective subjectivity associated with a prideful solidarism that was expressed in rituals of profound grief and loss, rage at the excessive punishment that the virus meted out to gay men, and the following out of both grief and rage in a radical activism directed at making the early drug treatment regime accessible to HIV-infected persons. As Kirsty Machon, a policy analyst for NAPWA at the time we did our fieldwork (2002–2003), has characterized it there was an 'epic quality' of that time: 'a time of heroes and many-headed monsters. A time when everything—but especially death—was larger than life itself' (Machon 2002, 1).

The current post-HAART era has been characterized by Dowsett (1996) as a 'post-AIDS' era.[3] There is no longer a unifying experience as these three statements, the first from Gary Dowsett (2006), an HIV social researcher, the second from Kirsty Machon (2002), a policy analyst working for NAPWA, and the third from Russell Westacott, Manager of Client Services at Australian AIDS Council of New South Wales (ACON)) represent:

[1] There is no single standpoint on AIDS anymore, not even among HIV+ people. There is no single standpoint on being gay or on gay

community anymore with which to build a singular community response to increased infection rates (Dowsett 2006, 10).

[2] It is sometimes hard ... to articulate what one might 'do' in response to HIV now that the epidemic has changed, and the virus does not have a universal narrative trajectory, that 'living with' is no longer a *de facto* political defiance to 'dying of', or a naming moment, a moment in which 'HIV' is given a face, a name, and a story to tell.

HIV has become both privatized and personalized, a set of stories struggling to be told. These stories are contingent, dependent, shaped and moulded by a thousand influences and congruencies. Luck. Genetics. The virus. Material circumstance. Sex and Love. Needles and rushes. Pharmokinetics. The mysteries of the organism (Kirsty Machon 2002, 4).

[3] Today, our service organizations are still central ports-of-call for many people living with HIV, but they are utilized primarily for service provision. For the most part, our service organizations are places that service consumers dip in and out of. These service consumers have ... found new dimensions to their lives, and they involve themselves less than they might have during previous times in the epidemic. The time when our organizations were strong congregating hubs that drew a diverse range of HIV+ people together for involvement in political and community activities, has passed.

This change in relationship has come about as more and more people living with HIV have less need to be full participants in the struggle to survive. Advances in medicines and sciences surrounding HIV mean that most people are doing quite well thank-you very much. It is probably fair to say that most people living with HIV are more worried about being able to keep their regular appointment with their GP for their three-monthly blood test than being involved in some type of community action, or even needing to find support from others living with HIV ... Increasingly people are finding their own personal strategies to live with HIV, that don't involve the need for regular contact with a service provider organization (Westacott, AFAO website 2008).

Thus in the 'post-AIDS' era, the collective subjectivity associated with the gay community's response to the epidemic has become more dispersed, differentiated, personalized and privatized. At the level of the individual person living with HIV a good deal of the management of the epidemic now takes place inside the practices of engagement as a patient working with a treatments doctor and the everyday aspects of managing the logistics of taking the drugs and dealing with their side-effects. The side-effects issue has loomed large so far in the post-HAART stage of the epidemic: as Race *et al.* put it in 2001 (1), 'the presence of effective but highly toxic treatments for HIV, which have a low tolerability but require an unusually high level of adherence, creates unique problems for those who prescribe them and are prescribed them'. Most of the drugs used cause nausea, vomiting and diarrhea, and one of the most difficult side effects associated with the protease inhibitors is lipodystrophy ('Lipo' in the vernacular) which causes fat accumulation in the abdomen along with a loss of tissue from the face, arms and legs. This affects especially HIV+ people who have spent a decade or so on antiviral drugs. One of them, David Menadue (2007), begins his article 'Lipo: any Progress?' with saying: 'For part of the past ten years I have felt I looked like a scarecrow. With my skinny arms and legs, bulging midriff, and sunken cheeks, at times I have looked a little scary or at best, a bit unusual'. As Menadue says, this has been 'a very stigmatizing condition, particularly when it affects the face … often "outing" people's HIV status to those around him whether they wish it or not'. He suggests that it 'seems likely that new generation antivirals will limit the chances of new HIV patients having to experience either the fat accumulation or fat loss, or at least to the same extent'. Of course these issues are under active negotiation between organized advocacy of gay men's interests such as NAPWA and the pharmaceutical companies.

Our fieldwork

Gary Dowsett, one of the authors of this chapter, is a social researcher in the HIV/AIDS field who has a background in the community-based politics of Gay Liberation. For this project, he had the standing and contacts to organize a workshop in Sydney in May 2002 that drew together two people working for the Australasian Society for HIV Medicine (ASHM), including its CEO, Levinia Crooks (whose permission to cite her by name we have obtained), two policy analysts working for NAPWA, two high case load HIV general practitioners, two social researchers working in the area, and an officer from the AIDS/Infectious Diseases Branch of New South Wales Health Department. Four members of the research team for this project were present at the workshop which was run by the two authors much like a focus group on current issues regarding HIV treatments. There were three follow-up interviews conducted by Anna Yeatman, one with Levinia Crooks, one with the two NAPWA policy analysts, and one with one of the two GPs. In addition to which, Anna Yeatman interviewed Kane Race, a researcher who has led much of the work on how the antiviral treatments stage of the epidemic emphasizes the importance of the clinical encounter taking account of quality of life issues for positive gay men. A number of related publications, some of which were community communications, were collected at this time. In May 2003, there was a day devoted to the project which brought together its reference group with other researchers including the two NAPWA policy analysts to contribute to discussion of peak bodies and their relationship to the development of service delivery-policy. Our discussion is limited to the Australian HIV epidemic as it has affected gay men. The informants for this case study are highly experienced and sophisticated participants in the clinical and social management of the epidemic. While it could be said that theirs is a 'Darlinghurst'-Sydney perspective, Darlinghurst being a point of concentration of the gay male community, the gay men living with HIV, and the headquarters of peak bodies such as NAPWA and ASHM, some of the workshop participants have extensive experience and/or research knowledge of the course of the epidemic in other Australian cities, regional and rural areas. That said the two high case load HIV GPs who were informants work in the Sydney context and, accordingly, when we use their discussion of the clinical encounter it is occurring in this context. In what follows we focus mostly on the field of medical service delivery and on how it has changed over the course of the epidemic's two stages: pre- and post-treatments.

Pre-treatments service delivery

With the advent of HAART, it can seem that there has been a 're-medicalization' of the epidemic. Yet as Levinia Crooks said in the workshop we organized: 'it's not really re-medicalization', it's always been medical, it's just that [in the pre-treatments stage] we couldn't treat it'. What remains constant is the positioning of the clinical management of the epidemic at a complex point of intersection and exchange between biomedical science and the lived experience of gay men, many of whom are identified with the gay community and its networks of communication (see Ariss, Dowsett and Carrigan 1995; Kippax and Race 2003). As Dowsett (1998, 182) put it: 'People living with HIV and AIDS fought vigorously for "living with", not "dying from", a claim to inclusion, to speaking for themselves, and to repositioning the patient as partner in disease management'. The lived experience of gay men refers not just to those who occupy the patient terms of the doctor/patient relationship but to also many of the general practitioners who were or are HIV specialists.

In this stage of the epidemic, the gay community was central to an organized response to the crisis. It was already politically mobilized and had been since the beginning of gay liberation in the early 1970s. Dowsett (1998, 179) reports that 'by the time of the first major Commonwealth [Government] initiatives in late 1984, the gay communities had already established the first HIV prevention activities (their major preoccupation over the next decade) and the first community-based, volunteer, home-care and support programmes for people living with HIV and AIDS'.

In her interview, Levinia Crooks described her experience with the epidemic going back to 1986. She said in her interview that she had a couple of close gay male friends, and so the epidemic was already an issue for her. At that time she was working in the Psychology Department at University of Wollongong, and she was part of a team that applied for New South Wales Health Department funding for research on HIV. The application centred on the development of psychosocial support for people with HIV, and it was successful. The team did interviews with 350 people living with HIV over three years, Levinia estimating that she did about 320 of these interviews. This research became the basis of the development of counseling services for both people living with HIV/AIDS and carers. She commented that with this kind of intensive and extensive research into the lived experience of the epidemic it was possible to provide a grounding for service delivery: 'by talking to a lot of people with HIV, and looking at how they behaved at the time, then we knew what was appropriate for them'. It was a time when relevant government agencies could not know how to respond to the epidemic without such research, so they were willing to give the researchers *carte blanche*, according to Crooks (interview data). Thus on the basis of this research it became possible to determine how best to manage the process of people receiving the HIV anti-body test, introduced in 1985, which established whether they were HIV+ or not: 'we got into the program of how counsellors were trained' and what a post-test counselling session should involve: 'that people should come back and see the doctor again, or even just the counsellor again, because what was coming out very clearly was people were being diagnosed and freaking out, basically' (interview data). Here we see how knowledge of the lived (gay) experience of the epidemic entered into the framing of clinical service delivery early. While at first there was a culture of silence and individual isolation in relation to post-test results, this broke in 1988 (Crooks 1989, 19) at the 3rd National Conference on AIDS. Crooks's comments about this shift are noteworthy:

> Keeping quiet about their infection had saved people from retribution, but it had obviously not provided the solutions, support and hope that speaking up was seen to provide. I use the word hope because that is what the small group of people who had been diagnosed for substantial periods of time did provide [they 'wore badges with the wording ALIVE AND VISIBLE']. Not hope that being a person living with AIDS was an easy task, not hope that suggested that the drugs were the answer to everything, not hope that said see you are going to live for ever. But the simple form of hope that said see, *I am a person like you, going through similar experiences, I am alive, I can share my experiences with you* and *I have a choice to fight or to give up*, or *I am not a useless, spent person*. This hope was also expressed through people with the virus taking on a voice and becoming active in the quest for information, treatment and services. As one person said *There may not be a cure yet, but I'm not going to stop fighting for the development of one* (Crooks 1989, 19, emphases in the original).

From this point on, Crooks suggests, the 'medico-scientific research fraternity', especially the medical scientists advising policy makers on the epidemiology of the epidemic, had to take notice of people with HIV-AIDS who 'demanded … to be talked with rather than just about' (Crooks 1989, 19).

Crooks also developed the first treatment education campaign aimed at positive people; this filled a gap at a time when post-diagnosis, positive people were ignored 'until they needed a carer' or hospitalization (interview data). ASHM was founded in 1990 as the peak body representing medical practitioners working in the HIV sector (over time, its membership has broadened to include health care workers and other graduates working in the HIV sector). Since joining the organization in the late 1990s, Crooks has become a central player in the development of ASHM, an organization that sustained her *modus operandi* as someone who entrepreneurs the development of an ongoing feedback loop between service delivery and research. In New South Wales, ASHM runs the accreditation program for prescribers of antiretrovirals. As of 2003, its membership base was 750, predominantly doctors, but also nurses, social workers, psychologists, community workers and policy people (interview data).

In the interview of a high case-load HIV general practitioner, who also participated in the workshop (and who is identified as GP#1) we get another set of glimpses into this stage of the epidemic. This is someone who trained in medicine in order to work in this area ('it was very clear that large amounts of people in my community were dying'), and who started practicing in 1989, interning for a year in the HIV ward at 'Vinnies' (Saint Vincent's Hospital in Darlinghurst), and then beginning in private practice. At this time GP#1 remembers that there was a strong sense of community uniting gay doctors with patients and with the community 'much more than ... now', and on being asked why, speculated 'I'm not sure that any of us thought we were doing this for a long time' (interview data). GP #1 added, 'But it just never ended'. Again in this set of stories the tight nexus between the clinical and lived aspects of the epidemic at least in this part of Sydney is evident. This doctor, as a medical student, lived in a gay household and recollects:

> ... we would get ... people knocking on the door all the time that we didn't know, whose partner had just been diagnosed with X or ... who'd just been given X diagnosis ... and had absolutely no ability to make head or tail of any of the information they were being given or what it meant ... So we used to spend a lot of time just digging out what various terms meant for people ...

In commenting further, GP#1 noted that there has been a huge change in the demands of doctors to explain things to patients over the last decade, certainly over the last five years: 'When I think back then ... there was still a hierarchy that doctors saw themselves in ... where they would waltz in, give a diagnosis and walk out, without any concept that in what they were actually telling one person, they were actually telling the other person'. Moreover, 'I mean ... telling one of the boys they were positive was actually telling the other boy they were positive', but they (the doctors) seemed to have a 'real lack of knowledge of gay relationships'.

At this point in a HIV career, this doctor's allegiance was 'to the patients and to the community'. On being asked about weathering the very difficult time when people were dying a lot (the period of the early 1990s up to about 1995) a very clear sense of this time of crisis was revealed:

> We used to have people dying at home that just refused to go to hospital. So it was not unusual for the practice to move. So people would turn up for an appointment except we'd be running the practice from somebody's house ... for a period of time. And people just dealt with it, I was always amazed that people dealt with it. So they'd come into the practice and the receptionist would give them their file and whatever else they needed and then they'd just come down and see me at whatever person's place it was.

In the workshop, this same doctor commented with reference to the current period of anti-retroviral treatments, 'just the luxury of actually having a six month [period of time] to talk about therapies with people', and then continued:

> When you think about it, it's really quite amazing. ... when we used to ... order death certificates in multiple books ... there was one period when Darlinghurst actually ran out of death certificates. ... it's a very different sort of perspective now.

Post-HAART service delivery

Now with the advent of antiretroviral drugs, HIV has been repositioned as 'a chronic manageable disease' (Rosengarten *et al.* 2000, 6). Yet it is not quite that simple as expressed eloquently by Robin Gorna (in Batrouney 1999, 6):

> I'm not convinced that what we've done is to move HIV to a chronic manageable condition. I think that what we've done is to give people more years of life, but not always very good years and essentially silenced people from expressing the complexity of what that is like. Time and time again in relation to HIV/AIDS you hear the phrase—'now that we have effective treatments', well my opinion is that these are lousy treatments. How can people approach going back to work when the side-effects of these treatments are physically and mentally debilitating?—that's not effective treatment.

At the workshop we conducted in 2002, the primary issue which came up regarding the contemporary drugs regime was side effects and their impact on quality of life. There was discussion of HIV-positive people choosing not to get treatment while still engaging in medical monitoring of their viral load thus permitting negotiation with their doctor as to what point of a low T-cell count they should start treatment ('if my T-cells go down below 350 with my next count, I agree I'll start treatments', as one of the HIV doctors contributed to the discussion).[4] There was also discussion of 'treatment breaks' either undertaken under medical supervision or on a self-medicating basis. The 'collaborative' nature of doctor-patient engagement fits Alison Moore's linguistic study of doctor-patient communication in HIV/AIDS health care based on 74 audio recordings of consultations between HIV doctors (mostly general practitioners) and patients in and around Sydney in the period 1995–1997. Moore (2005, 103) reports: 'A key finding was that doctors and patients in HIV medicine often construe the agency of one participant as a resource for the agency of another rather than competing with the agency of the other'.

Uncertainty dogs this field of service delivery. The science, the drugs, the virus itself, along with the lived experience of the infection constitute a complex, interpenetrating set of dynamic, mobile horizons. At the same time, within the clinical encounter, there can be no way of scientifically settling just what kind of trade-off between effective treatment and patient quality of life should be achieved. This has to be a matter of highly individualized negotiation between doctor and patient.

At the time of conducting our workshop in May 2002, the *HIV Futures 3* survey of positive Australians was just about to be released and a number of workshop participants already knew its findings. So it is relevant to indicate that, at that time, of the 894 HIV+ Australians surveyed (not just gay men), 38.4% report experiencing lipodystrophy, 30.7% weight loss, 68.5% low energy or fatigue, 52.2% have a sleep disorder, 33.8% confusion or memory loss; of the total, 71.7% are currently using antiretroviral (ARV) treatments, while 86.9% have used ARV at some time; and 41.3% of those currently on ARV have taken a break from ARV therapy, mostly for a combination of lifestyle and clinical reasons, with doctors less likely to be consulted before a break than afterward, while 67.1% saw their doctor during a treatment break (Grierson *et al.* 2002, vii–ix).

There was some interesting discussion of the issue of the treatments/quality-of-life conundrum at the workshop. Here is one where Levinia Crooks and GP #1 are participating:

Levinia: ... we had that long period of time where basically GPs provided palliative care. There wasn't a lot of other options ... Then we had antiretrovirals ... Did we push 'treat hard, treat early, treat lots' as a sort of active response to now, we've got something, let's go out there and do it?

GP #1: ... the only reason we moved back from 'hit it all the time' is—

Levinia: (and another male voice): Is because of toxicity.

GP #1: ... It's still an infectious disease. If we had non-toxic, low side-effect therapies, we'd all still use them from the beginning, the entire time.

Just how 'empowered' a patient can be in this situation was also discussed. Early on in the workshop Levinia Crooks observed, 'there's an additional dilemma, which is the rhetoric around HIV ... has been since about 1987 trying to empower the infected person to make decisions, and now when ... people are making decisions to not treat, or to interrupt treatment, there's somehow this thing where you're saying "but you're not meant to make *that* decision"'. Here is another discussion sequence that indicates something of the complexity of these issues. It occurs in context of a discussion of someone with ten T-cells who decides not to go onto treatments which means he is likely to die.

GP #1: I am actually not convinced that ... the boy with ten T-cells is making it [a decision] on the basis of any information at all ... They don't understand what's actually going to be involved in this process ...

HIV social researcher #1: That's a way of coping as well sometimes. You're prepared to think about the endpoint which is being dead but you don't necessarily want to go into all the ...

GP #1 (over these last words): They're not prepared to think about it ... that's actually not really gonna happen in any sort of nasty or difficult way. It's just gonna be an instantaneous thing. One day they're gonna be alive, exactly as they are now, and the next day they'll be dead. And there is no process of actually how that's gonna occur.

HIV social researcher #1: But maybe the way of dealing with that is just by taking one day at a time. ... different people [have] ... different ways of dealing with the illness ... And if I were somebody with ten T-cells that came to you and said, look I don't really want to think about all that messy stuff about how I'm gonna die, but I know I'm going to die and it's probably going to be, you know, in the next few months. And you really strongly try to convince me otherwise and talk me out of that, I might feel like that was disempowering—

GP #1: Well yeah, I mean—and patronizing.

GP #1: ... I mean I think that you know the idea that it's empowering somehow to actually make a decision and avoid information ... on the basis of actually not knowing any of the ways that the things will occur, I find bizarre. It's not empowering.

HIV social researcher #1: Because choosing not to know can, maybe what you know is that getting that information is going to push you in one particular direction so powerfully that you don't want to go, that the only choice you have is not to know in the first place.

GP #1: But part of the process of what I have to do as a clinician right is actually make people look at that. ... If I've got a person who ... comes to me and says, ... I understand this is how it's going to be, and these are all the things I've got in place, and this is how I actually want to go. I'm fine with that. I don't have a problem with that. My point is that they hadn't thought it through and they're actually not accepting that as some sort of empowering decision in the way that you're saying.

This same doctor when interviewed also expressed concern about treatment resistance which occurs when people take their drugs badly. GP #1 expressed frustration at not being able to be direct in advising patients that 'You have got X number of choices left. If you blow 'em like this you've got a year and a half worth of therapy and that's it'. In the workshop there was an interesting exchange between the two GPs regarding the point at which they might refuse to continue treatments of a non-adhering patient:

GP #1: ... at what point [do] we actually pull back ... and say, no, I'm not writing any more scripts because you are ... actually creating self harm in doing this? ... when I've done that, when I've actually refused to write prescriptions for patients or ... terminated the relationship, I've actually thought that's a very interesting area and ... a lot of the time it hasn't quite led to where I thought it was going to lead. It's actually changed the nature of the relationship ... [the patient says] I didn't realize it was so serious, right? ...

GP #2: I suppose my experiences where I've terminated a relationship have been similar in that ... it sometimes makes you as a clinician much more desirable to the patient. And [laughs] they very much want to pursue that relationship and it changes the balance, and it certainly individualizes the relationship. I mean it's not something that one does very often.

Adding to the complexity of the relationship between these GPs and their patients is any doctor's engagement with his or her patients as a clinical researcher. We did not get much information about this aspect of the engagement although GP #2 commented:

... if we're honest, doctors rely on patients ... as clinical research subjects, to get funding, to get kudos within their own community, to publish papers, to talk at conferences. So there are whole other issues involved in that relationship. And sometimes patients see those other relationships and are suspicious of [them]. On the other hand, for the patient sometimes it's the only way they can access the newest, latest therapy or what seems to be potentially the newest, latest and best therapy.

In interview, GP #1 suggested that the vital role the high-load HIV-GPs play in clinical trials is unique in contemporary medicine, and it gives these GPs more professional leverage than normal in relation to the medical specialists in this field (the infectious disease specialists and immunologists).

Both of these high HIV case-load, Sydney-based GPs were identified with the gay community and saw themselves as advocates for their patients. While this did not displace their sense of medical professionalism and responsibility, they had no difficulty accepting the importance of working with the lived experience of the disease on the part of their individual patients. This is clearly evident in how GP #2 spoke of preparing an individual to start antiretroviral therapy:

A good analogy ... is with diabetes. If you look at a young person with ... type one diabetes they're going to be on insulin for the rest of their lives or they're gonna die—early. And you have real compliance issues with young people with diabetes. Adherence is really hard and managing the blood sugars is really hard, and ... they're at that stage where they're really resistant to authority figures and all the rest of it. ... but the bottom line, if they go through a rough track and they start using their insulin again, they're going to be fine, unless they've knocked off a kidney or something. Whereas when you start looking at people with HIV and going through that process with them of negotiating starting therapy, sometimes it would take me six months to negotiate them commencing therapy because I didn't want them to start therapy until they understand completely what it means to be on therapy. What the risks to them are if they stop and start and are non-adherent, in terms of resistance and future drugs. Sometimes I'll spend six months of seeing this person to ... get to the stage where I think they're ready to start treatment so that they will be adherent and they'll have ... ten, 15, 20 years out of that therapy. Whereas if someone starts therapy when they don't really want to ... they stop it or they just take one a day instead of three ... Eighteen months down the track ... they're suddenly resistant to three drugs and—

The same GP commented later in the workshop about this process of preparation: 'That's not changing scientific boundaries, that's a skill that I've learned that's peculiar to HIV medicine'.

It is clear that neither of these GPs practiced what Race *et al.* (2001, 9) call 'the consumer formulation' of the clinical encounter, one where 'the doctor's skills are portrayed as a commodity or service which patients can elect to make use of, by means of "informed choice"'. Instead both assumed a pedagogical responsibility for teaching the patient how to engage effectively and responsibly with the drug treatment regime while simultaneously maintaining awareness of the impact of taking these drugs on the patient's lived experience and life world. In terms of the two general styles of HIV general practice that Race *et al.* suggest are characteristic of this type of medical practice, these two individual doctors seem to fit the first one that they mention:

Of the many approaches to the patient's world we have encountered in this research, two general styles are worth outlining ... The first places a very high importance on adherence to HAART, and takes a proactive approach with respect to aspects of patients' lives felt to inhibit adherence. The second treats the patients' world more liberally, and tends not to take on matters that concern patients' lives beyond those amenable to medical solutions. Both of these general styles have advantages, and both have certain weaknesses. For example, while the first may appear overly intrusive, and sometimes dismissed the lived realities of treatment, practitioners who adopted it were more fluent in the historical, lived, and particular conditions affecting their patients, and had developed pragmatic techniques to help patients overcome some of these. Though the second approach accords much respect to the priorities and values of the patient, and may acknowledge the specificity of values that inform medicine, at times it can produce a reluctance to engage patients in evaluation or working on certain aspects of their worlds (Race *et al.* 2001, 3).

The relationship of the clinical setting to a wider context of HIV service delivery

In the pre-HAART stage of the epidemic, as already argued, there was an embedding of the doctor-patient relationship within community-based service delivery of various kinds: counselling, post-diagnosis education, prevention education, caring circles, and so on. From 1996 onwards such embedding has been becoming not so evident even though the major AIDS advocacy organizations continue to play a vital role in treatments education and advocacy (with the pharmaceuticals and policy makers). This is a complex topic that involves a number of factors including the way in which the epidemic has been personalized at the level of the individual living with HIV. In terms of the personalization of the epidemic, it is the individual living with HIV who is the key player integrating the clinical encounter with both the pharmacy and his life world in which the virus and the logistics of treating it play out (for a detailed analysis of these logistics see Race and Wakeford 2000). It's also the case that as Levinia Crooks suggested in interview, 'the time of the group has passed'. She commented further of individuals living with HIV:

> ... I don't need to talk about HIV as the only thing I talk about all the time. I want to get on with life. ... because it was so consuming for such a period for so many people, and so many people were dying, and it was a ... reality of this could happen to me next week, sort of thought. Because people would get sick quickly, y'know. Fine today, PCP next week, in hospital, dead, boom. Fine today, find a lump, yes

it's lymphoma, yes it's treatment, treatment doesn't work, lymphoma gets bigger, person goes to hospital, person dies. Three months. ... then there was a lot of talking and ... for many people with HIV it was all of their lives. ... So ... I think it's a reaction against that ...

At the same time a number of participants at the workshop, including Levinia Crooks, suggested that there should be more non-medical service delivery focused on toxicity, treatment breaks, and, also, discussion of the non-rational aspects of patient engagement with the challenges of living with both the disease and the current treatments regime. Regarding the latter, two of the workshop participants were most interested in the need of patients to have their anxiety, abjection and need for reassurance acknowledged. Arguably such needs cannot be accommodated within the medical model of information-based problem solving. This area of need fits the emphasis of John Daye (2001, 3), in his address to the 2001 8th National Conference of People Living With HIV/AIDS on the need to provide psycho-therapeutic and counselling services to positive people: 'There is a paucity of services and facilities to effectively deal with mental health and emotional/psychological health issues that are specific to positive people's needs'.

Notwithstanding treatments optimism, dying from this disease is still part of the picture even though just how it is part of the picture is much less certain than in the pre-treatments stage of the pandemic. As GP #2 commented in the workshop, 'the dying's always in the [doctor's] room, but it's often left out'. In interview, Levinia Crooks remarked on this topic:

LC: What used to happen was ... sort of an acceptance of, okay, there ain't a lot more that can happen here, I'm on the way out ... There was a knowledge that this is not gonna get better ... and it might get worse ... Now there's this ... [whirring sound]

AY: Just for the tape, that was sort of jagged circles.

LC: That means people are sort of ... sliding down a razor blade of life but it's a really long razor blade ... the challenge is there for long periods of time.

AY: I was really struck by our workshop ... by the lack of talking about this ... it was a very rational decision-making model type workshop that we worked with ... yes the theme of abjection came up, but there was nothing in-between. The lived experience of the now wasn't being reported. So does that mean there's not much talking happening? And why is that?

LC: I don't think people want to burst the bubble.

AY: ... the belief that the treatments might work ... yet people know they won't work ...

LC: Ah, but they believe ... there's another one around the corner ...

AY: ... but ... the overload on someone's system of these very complex drug cocktails is going to have consequences.

LC: Yeah, but what if intergraze [inhibitors, a new drug] don't have the same impact?

AY: But if someone has been on these drug regimes it's not like they're starting from scratch.

LC: No ... But there are people who are going onto new drugs and there's only 12,000 people infected, they'll be dead sooner or later. That might sound horrid but it's [true] ... Maybe the people who've only been on treatment for four years have got the capacity to reverse that. Maybe treatment breaks are going to be the thing that'll enable people to stay on toxic treatments longer. There's all of these reasons for hope that cause people not to have this discussion.

This very human need to continue to hope, and to have others 'hold hope' for oneself (on this see Flaskas 2007, 33), begins to explain something of the subtleties and complexities that face any service organization that seeks to address the contemporary lived experience of the epidemic. Moreover, the uncertainties surrounding the moving train of the virus, the science, the drug treatments, their course over time and their impact on individuals' embodied experience of the infection, makes it difficult to know how the community service sector might address these issues, as is evident in the following workshop exchange between Levinia Crooks and one of the HIV social researchers:

LC: On a service provision level ... the community sector has withdrawn itself from providing service and I think part of that has happened because there has been the advent of treatment, the medical-isation or remedicalisation of HIV by the community sector, the placement of the management of that person in the clinical setting. And then now what we're seeing is that that is a really difficult thing to sustain. That toxicity is making that not a sufficient solu-tion. And yet the community sector in my opinion hasn't kept up with how it does the work to support making that more sustainable.

HIV social researcher #2: The moment that treatments information hit [the] Vancouver [1996 International AIDS Conference], the com-munity sector was irretrievably on the back foot. ... it's never been able to keep up with the information flow ever since. To participate in increasing and ever-spiralling amount, change, speed, changeabil-ity—all those characteristics that constitute pharmacological and treatments information now. ... it's not I would argue the role of the community sector. ... The role is actually to interfere in the pace of information flow so that people can think about what's going on. In other words, to engage in social acts of communication. One of them is to support the people who are providing the information and decision-making, in clinical settings, i.e. doctors ...

LC: ... clearly the community has a role ... but distancing itself from ... the epidemic is not ... the way to go about fulfilling it.

HIV social researcher #2: No but ... you don't do it around HIV is my next step. This community you do it around gayness and self care.

LC: I think we've got a real difficulty about even the construction of what is community ... We're talking about a limited bit of commu-nity that's relatively close to here [Darlinghurst] that's ... predom-inantly gay male, white, educated and reads. ... But if you look outside of that group, I think there's very little applicability for what we've been talking about.

HIV social researcher #1: I think [name of HIV social researcher #2] is right ... community has been on the back foot since 1996. And is still kind of locked into this rather unproductive struggle with science and clinical medicine ... over ... who has ... the best cap-acity in a sense to provide certain types of information. When I think Anna's question ... is a really interesting one what is the community's relationship toward this non-rational stuff?

This concern about gay community and its place has been ever-present and ever-changing as an ongoing dynamic in the Australian experience of its HIV epidemic (see Rowe and Dowsett 2008). Over the 26 years of HIV/AIDS, this dynamic has not just shaped how the epidemic has been handled in Australia, but contributed significantly to shifts in health policy in other areas.

Conclusion

General practice medicine in relation to the HIV/AIDS epidemic in the gay male community has always been highly individualized but it also has taken place in a dynamic gay cultural context that has produced veterans of the politically mobilized response of the gay community to the epidemic in Australia. It offers a rare glimpse into the historical and ongoing dynamic of the intersections between clinical practice, medical research, the development of new pharmaceutical products, and the lived experience of people living with a chronic and fatal disease at a particular point of time in a particular place. This case study also reveals how contingent the individualization of service delivery in a clinical setting is on a range of 'external' forces which in turn interact with shifts and changes in clinical practice. A second feature is the velocity of change in a phenomenon like HIV/AIDS, where overnight technological advances in Australia and internationally can alter the dynamics of the relationships between all the players, elevating the medical practitioner at one moment, the activist at another, various collectivities (ASHM and its membership, the gay community, government, etc.)—sometimes even the patient—while robbing others of prominence. A third feature is the professionalizing of the players in this sector. Not only are the HIV GPs clustered around special prescribing rights and an organization like ASHM, but so too are those directly affected by HIV/AIDS in NAPWA, and those politically and socially involved in AFAO. These collectivities have been participating in the policy development and delivery process as partners, as protesters and activists, and as stakeholders since the beginning of the Australian epidemic. The ongoing development of the national HIV/AIDS strategy (and State/Territory policies) to govern and direct the provision of services to those affected by HIV/AIDS is a central underlying feature of individualized service delivery in this area. These policy and program management components of clinical care are far more obvious to the individual PLWHA than it might be to, say, a person suddenly suffering a stroke. In this way, the tragedy that is HIV/AIDS has contributed to a remarkable 'opening-up' of the health system and the medical world in its 26 year history, and the story is not over.

Notes

1 The prominence of gay community organizations in the management of the epidemic 'is not surprising when one considers that 86.9% of cumulative AIDS cases in Australia are related to "male homosexual contact" with and without injecting drug use, and male-to-male sexual transmission of HIV is involved in 81.0% of cumulative HIV infections and 84.8% of incident infections each year (Dowsett 2003, 122)'. These proportions have remained relatively stable throughout the Australia epidemic to date.
2 For the current strategy see Commonwealth of Australia (2005) *National HIV/AIDS Strategy: Revitalising Australia's Response 2005–2008*.
3 For further discussion of this concept see also Dowsett and McInnes (1996), Dowsett *et al.* (2000) and Dowsett (2006).
4 'HIV is constantly multiplying within the body. The amount of virus being reproduced can be indicated by the viral load. Viral load measurements are taken by a blood test ... The higher the result the greater the amount of viral reproduction, and the greater likelihood of damage to the immune system. The immune system is made up of a lot of different types of cells. HIV targets a group of these cells called T-cells (also known as CD4 cells) which protect you from bugs or germs you may come in contact with. A normal range of T-cells is between 500 and more than 1,200. Current medical guidelines recommend anti HIV treatment if a person has 500 or less CD4 cells or a viral load of more than 10,000 copies (from Batrouney and Crooks 1998, no pagination)'.

12
Facilitating Independence and Self-determination: The Case of a Disability Employment Service

Anna Yeatman

Introduction

The conduct of the service delivery relationship between service user and service agency determines whether service delivery is both individualized and effective from the user's point of view. The service delivery relationship is democratic when the service user's voice and, as appropriate, choice are given the central role in determining the direction, pacing, and outcomes of this relationship. Our focus here is on contractualist protocols for democratizing the conduct of the service delivery relationship. These are protocols that provide structure and focus for the relationship in such as way as to ensure that there is dialogue and negotiation between the service user and the service worker.

In turning our focus to the *conduct* of the service delivery relationship, our emphasis is deliberate. It is an emphasis on the governance of the service delivery relationship for this is more central to the possibilities and actualities of this relationship than the good will and skills of individual service workers. This emphasis also characterizes the individualized care planning structure of governance in the Looking After Children initiative (see Chapter 9). A highly skilled worker who is a committed and strategic advocate for service users can learn 'to work the system', but their effectiveness as a worker depends on the institutional design of the service into which their work fits. If such institutional design does not invite and support them in working effectively and democratically with a service user, they cannot make up for this deficit by their own dedication and skills.

The conduct of the service delivery relationship is of consequence when service delivery is undertaken as a relationship that extends over a relatively long period of time and where the service can make a real difference to the service user's quality of life and/or life chances. In what follows we emphasize the role of the service agency in designing and implementing a structure for the conduct of the service delivery relationship that is contractualist in character. The freedom of the agency to do this, when it is dependent on government funding, is constrained by government policy and funding regime. Government may or may not facilitate a service agency's interest in democratic design for the conduct of the service delivery relationship. This turned out to be an issue in our case study of a specialist employment service for people with mental illness described shortly.

Design issues for the democratization of the service delivery relationship

Within the relationship, is the consumer/user respected and valued as an individual? Does the consumer feel that service staff accept him or her as the person s/he is? Is his/her autonomy cultivated and enabled by service staff? Do service staff explain things clearly, and provide information of the kinds that enable the service user to think well about his or her options? And, finally, if the service is of a kind that makes the relationship between service user and service staff the key to whether the service is delivered effectively, then does service management and staff give careful attention to how this relationship is structured, developed and maintained?

It is the service relationship between individual worker and individual consumer that is the foundation of effective service delivery in cases where the nature of the service depends on creative interaction and complex communication between these two parties. By creative interaction, we mean that service design positions both individuals so that they draw upon their respective strengths in the interaction. By complex communication, we mean that the two individuals are able to talk about matters that are difficult, sensitive and emotionally charged for the consumer, and, that thereby, the consumer becomes more aware of his or her needs and wants. Where the service relationship functions like this, there is likely to be a degree of intimacy between worker and consumer and, following on from this, a reciprocity of gift exchange where the nature of the gift concerns how each uses and gives of his/her self.

Take three instances where the service relationship is the key to service effectiveness. The simplest is personal care, where in order to be transferred from bed to chair (or toilet or shower), an individual, whose disability does not permit him/her to do this him/herself, has to depend on the assistance of a paid worker. The paid worker can work with the individuality of this person or disregard it. If the latter, the person will feel s/he is being treated as a thing and s/he will feel profoundly vulnerable and powerless, regardless of the degree of skill the worker brings to the operation. The transfer is an entirely different phenomenon when the worker engages in a dialogical partnership with this individual and listens to him or her as the expert on how best to move him or her. The routine of this transaction then is flexibly adapted to how the service user and worker present themselves and work together on any particular day. The worker's acknowledgment of the service user as an individual who may or may not have had a bad night, who may be excited about something that is about to happen, and the interchanges this acknowledgment involves, are where exchange of self occurs. Thus, the nature of the service may be fairly simple, but its delivery is not only relatively complex but entirely dependent on the quality of the relationship that is achieved by both service worker and service user. Usually it is service workers, plural, because someone who needs daily transfer assistance will need the support of a team of workers. Given the centrality of the quality of a relationship with a team of workers that is built over time to the quality and effectiveness of the service, it is important that service providers do all that they can to ensure continuity in these relationships if they are working for the consumer.

The second instance is a teaching and learning relationship, whether this is in a school setting or in a university supervision relationship. It is impossible for anyone to do significant new learning without changing who they are. This is a difficult thing to do under any circumstance. It requires both courage and a sense of safety in respect of the context in which one is developing and changing. Such courage and safety are facilitated by a teacher who supplies the recognition of what this process means to the individual, provides encouragement, advice, and, as needed, instruction. The effective teacher also 'holds the space' within which the student is developing and growing by being attentive to the student's needs for carefully paced and supported learning within a delimited spatial and temporal environment that supports such learning. In this respect the teacher provides an equivalent of what Donald Winnicott called, in relation to the psychoanalytic setting of the clinical relationship, 'the facilitating environment'.

The third instance is the kind of service our case study involves. This is the provision of employment services to people who are mentally ill, where the service involves employment counselling and employment-related life planning, job search and placement, job site training and advocacy, job maintenance support and follow-up (see Danley and Mellen 1987). This type of service has much in common with a teaching and learning relationship. An individual who has a mental illness has to feel accepted, respected, safe and supported in risking engagement in employment. It may not be the right time for this person to be attempting employment, and if this is the case, s/he needs to be supported and facilitated in making this decision, and thus exiting the service in such a way that re-entry further down the track is an option. Even if an individual is unable to achieve employment, or to keep employment at a particular time, their engagement with the service can be positive in enhancing their sense of self-worth and their ability to learn to manage their illness. It is only through the development of a capacity to learn to live with and manage their illness that the individual with an ongoing mental illness can live within the world and attempt to live a normal life. It is the service worker's acceptance, encouragement and skilling of this individual, and the relationship between the two, that are the key to whether this type of service can be successfully transacted. Success depends on an individual consumer developing his or her self-knowledge and self-esteem, and making the courageous leap of faith that is involved in hoping that things can get better for him or her.

Relational contracting in service delivery

As proposed above, the quality and the effectiveness of the service are not independent of how the service relationship is transacted and, more broadly, conducted. It is for this reason that contractualist protocols assume an importance in providing structure for the relationship as it is transacted over time. Our proposition in this paper is that contract in service delivery is a fundamental component of client-centred service delivery in cases where the conduct of the service delivery relationship over time is central to the effectiveness of service delivery.

Let us turn now to justifying our use of the language of contract in this context. We have no doubt that our description of negotiated agreements within the service delivery relationship as contractual in character is correct. Contract of this kind has a genealogy that can be traced to both social work use of the language of contract, and to learning contracts in education settings.

Contractualism of this kind is a case of what legal theorists call relational contracting; it is to be distinguished from the classical legal doctrine of contract that was distilled in nineteenth century common law. On this conception, contract is a legally enforceable exchange of promises (Yeatman 1998b, 230). It involves a discrete transaction where the terms of the contract concern primarily the conditions of entry and exit to the relationship.

Some legal theorists argue that even in the case of contract that conforms to the classical legal model, the legal understanding of contract does not capture the way in which the parties to a contract see it. Alain Roy (2001, 5), for example, suggests that:

> Far from languishing in the back of a drawer, contracts act as a referential platform, or relationship guide, to which the parties refer to orient their actions based on expectations and aspirations that each of them has expressed. In short contracting parties do not view their contract through the same lens that lawyers use. The coercive function is relegated to a secondary role.

In this connection, Roy (2001, 5) cites the work of the legal scholar, Ian Macneil, who proposes that '[Performance planning'] is, after all, the way most participants view most contract planning—only lawyers and other trouble-oriented folk look to contracts primarily as a source of trouble and disputation, rather than as a way of getting things done.' The way participants view contract planning is in fact closer to the idea of relational contracting—developed by Macneil and other legal theorists (see also Gordon 1985)—than it is to the classical legal conception of contract.

Macneil developed the idea of relational contracting in the context of distinguishing between (a) contracts that fall into the category of a discrete transaction, involving 'no significant relationship between the parties beyond the exchange of consents'; and (b) contracts that fall into the category of 'relational' exchanges, these being 'a project in which the parties intend to cooperate over the long-term (Roy 2001, 6)'. Thus, legal theorists have applied the idea of relational contracting to intimate relationships of cohabitation and/or close personal relationships (Roy 2001; Kingdom 2000; Wightman 2000). Kingdom (2000, 20) represents the relational contract:

> The relational contract ... is one which forms a relationship between the parties which extends over time, which is concomitant with and

integrates with the parties' other activities, which is more flexible, and which may be renegotiated in the light of the parties' changing circumstances.

Defined in this way, relational contracting has much in common with contractualist protocols for the conduct of the service delivery relationship that we discuss here. Legal theorists who are interested in relational contracting, however, have neglected the use of contract in service delivery.[1]

Contract in service delivery is *infra*-legal rather than legal in character although the normative expectations that inform it may have a basis in legislation and policy mandate for publicly funded service agencies as is true of the case we discuss. It has a degree of formality, and there is, as we shall see, a paper trail for agreements that are negotiated between the service worker and the consumer. But this type of contract is not a binding exchange of promises. Rather it is a flexible tool for eliciting mutual agreement between the parties and for structuring the development of their ongoing interaction. Attention to *infra*-legal contractualist protocols of the kind that interest us here may throw light on what the legal theorists are attempting to think about by way of relational contracting. Whether they do or not, they are worth attention in their own right.

The case study

In this article, the empirical reference is to a case study of a specialist employment service working with individuals with a psychiatric disability in Sydney over the period 1998–2000. This is an 'open' or in US language 'competitive' employment service meaning it is intended to prepare individuals for employment in the regular labour market. In Australia, at that time, the disability programs branch of the federal government Family and Community Services agency funded services of this kind. Since we undertook the case study the policy environment of this kind of service has changed. In fact it was changing as we did the case study. Now, in contrast to the period we studied, the program orientation for the service is clearly 'welfare to work', the policy department responsible for open employment is the Department of Employment and Workplace Relations, and the funding basis of this type of service has shifted from a block grant to an individualized, performance-oriented funding system. The change in policy environment is sufficiently radical as to make it unlikely that the democratic approach to service delivery discussed here could be sustained, but of course this is a matter for further empirical enquiry (although for some suggestion on this front, see Peter Saunders 2005).

We undertook interviews with the service manager, the senior employment consultant, several of the employment consultants, and three service clients in addition to examining relevant documents bearing on the work of the service including its internal policy guidelines. We also got access, with their consent, to two clients' files. All names of people involved in our case study have been changed and no identifying information has been used in our reportage on them.

Our description of the contractualist protocols in this service was shared with the service management and workers, and they took the opportunity to comment on and to correct it. The same draft of this paper was presented in March 2001 to a regional conference of the Australian Association for Competitive Employment, the peak body for specialist open employment services working mostly with people who have intellectual and/or psychiatric disabilities. The feedback from these provider representatives was that the empirically based section of the paper accurately captured their practice and client-centred ethos.

We turn now to the empirically based analysis of contractualist protocols in this type of service setting after first briefly describing the service agency. In the final section of this paper, we consider the limits of contract in democratizing the service delivery relationship, before we briefly conclude by returning to the issue of what kind of governmental funding and management regime either facilitates or hinders contractualist service delivery.

The service agency

The service agency began in 1994 with funding from the Commonwealth Government. It provides employment counselling to two categories of people—people with intellectual disability, and people with mental illness—that is designed to prepare and skill them to enter regular, paid employment. Until subjected to the new regime of welfare to work, the value orientation of the service was shaped by legislative and wider policy discourse of disability rights that came into existence with the Disability Services Act of 1986. Services funded under this Act had to comply with Disability Service Standards. This agency was noteworthy when we studied it in 1998–2000 for the reflection in its service policy and procedures of a thorough integration of its own quality assurance protocols (including regular service-initiated auditing and use of a yearly consumer survey to give feedback to the service) with the legislation and Commonwealth Government Disability Service Standards. Now that the service comes under the Department of Employment and Workplace Relations (DEWR) it is subject to a more generic set of expectations concerning performance and contract management 'similar to that used for the highly successful Job Network programme (DEWR *Annual Report 2004–2005*, p. 3)'.

Contractualist protocols in client-centred service delivery

The role of contractualist protocols in service delivery is to build the agency of the individual client into the service transaction. These protocols are contractualist because they function on behalf of making the service delivery relationship subject to a process of negotiated agreement between service deliverer and client. In this way, the relationship is mediated by the individualized consent of the client. It is what Yeatman (1998) calls the ethos of contemporary contractualism.

Contractualism of this kind has the feature of mutual agreement in common with legal and economic contracts. However, unlike legal and economic contracts, it does not require the fiction that the parties to the agreement are equals. Moreover, service delivery contractualism presupposes that the asymmetry in the relationship originates in the worker's capacity to give a service to an individual that s/he cannot reciprocate.

In addition, it is not an exchange that is based in self-interest, as this term is usually understood. In the worker's case, self-interest in terms of having a reasonably secure, good, and decently paid job operates of course. But self-interest in this sense does not enter into the worker's commitment to giving a service that a client finds to be useful and important. As we found in our interviews with workers, their commitment to good service can be at their personal expense as in, for example, the development of burn out.[2] Moreover, they do not get what they think they should be paid for this work, and it is below what salaried professionals with their degree of experience and education would be paid in other sectors.[3] On the client's side, it is his or her self-interest in establishing a more independent life through employment that brings him or her to the service. However, there may be major issues of motivation and clarification of achievable goals that s/he has to tackle with the support of the worker if s/he is to take advantage of what the service has to offer. The client's wants, in other words, become clarified in a dialogical process of search after what is possible and achievable by way of employment and maybe further training and education options. To engage in such a process of clarification, the client has to accept the gift of service commitment to him or her that the worker offers. The vulnerability of this client group (people with a mental illness), and the importance of the development of a trust relationship between workers and clients comes out in the following exchange. The exchange is between us, the service manager, the senior employment consultant, and one of the workers in the feedback session on the draft of this paper. The reference to protocols is elaborated in the next section.

> *Researcher*: Clients appear vulnerable. I'm not sure we've brought this out in our papers. There's the stigma (in relation to disclosure [of mental illness]). [And] they seem to experience a loss of trust in themselves in both their capacity to be cognitively competent and also in terms of confidence. Is this right?

> *Service manager*: Yes. That comes out clearly in the [annual consumer] survey [that the service conducts].

> *Employment Consultant #1:* On the Vocational Profile [Protocol #5] which lists barriers to employment, some will say 'all of them', or pick about six.

> *Service Manager*: Our success is due to such things as the Vocational-Personal Profile [Protocols #5 and 6] which allows us to get to know the individuals. This humanises the process. A lot of services start with the IEP [the Individual Employment Plan, Protocol #10]. In these cases there is no time to paint a picture of the individual.

> *Senior Employment Consultant* [who is the direct manager of the staff working with this client group]: A lot of services start with a clinical focus on illness. However, what makes a person vulnerable is that while they might want to work, they don't understand the consequences of that for themselves. We discuss this with them. This comes from there being a *trust* relationship between staff and clients.

> *Service Manager*: We explore the relationship between a willingness to work and the motivation to do it on a day-to-day basis.

The contractualist protocols that are used in this service are listed in Table 12.1. It represents the formal face of these protocols as they are

Table 12.1   The formal aspect of contractualist protocols at a specialist disability employment service

Referral	**1. Referral Form** To be filled out, signed and dated by client—contact details; diagnosis; whether receiving support from another employment service; whether registered with the Government income support agency; which type of benefit client is receiving; contact person. Plus 'confirmation of diagnosis' to be filled out and signed by doctor/case manager.
Process of Entry	**2. Service Information Handbook** Covers: (a) information about the service—these include the development of an individual employment plan for each person accepted by the service that is realistic and reflects the person's choices; (b) what the client's rights are; (c) the client's responsibilities; (d) what to do if the client has a complaint; (e) how will privacy and confidentiality be handled.
	3. Acknowledgment of Receipt of Handbook A statement that the client signs/dates along with his/her employment consultant (EC) to say s/he has received a copy of the handbook, has read it and/or has had it explained, and has understood the sections on his/her rights, including right to privacy and confidentiality; and what to do if not happy with the service.
	4. Authority to Release/Gain Information A statement that client signs/dates to give the service the authority to get (on a need to know basis) information about him/her from his/her doctor/case manager/family, and to release anonymous statistical information to relevant government agencies. The actual consent is 'to release and/or gain any information relevant to my involvement with the organisation' and the signature comes on a line after the statement 'I, the undersigned, can at any time change or cancel this authority'.
Assessment Process	**5. Vocational Profile** A detailed diagnostic tool for identification of the individual's vocational aspirations, preferred working hours and conditions, employment goals for next 12 months, identification of how work will impact on his/her life, skills and employment background, and a review of his/her employment experience, strengths, and difficulties.

Table 12.1   The formal aspect of contractualist protocols at a specialist
disability employment service – *continued*

	6. **Personal Profile** A detailed assessment tool that covers personal details, educational background, employment and voluntary work histories, mental health history and current situation, support network, and impact of disability (e.g. sleeping, side effects of medication, etc), present living arrangement, hobbies and interests, issues of concern.
	7. **Agreed Disclosure Authority** Client signs and dates a form that elicits clear information about whether s/he wants to disclose and for what kinds of employment position.
	8. **Ongoing Health Strategy** The equivalent of a living will for what an individual client wants the service to do if s/he becomes ill—covers who to contact, what does s/he want to do about his/her job. Also asks client to identify warning signs for recurrence of his/her illness. And statement that if service considers his/her health or that of others is at risk, service reserves the right to contact the appropriate organizations. Signed off/dated by both the client and his/her EC.
Job Search and Maintaining Employment Processes	9. **Individual Employment Plan (IEP)** Four pages: P1 covers vocational achievements, present employment details if applicable. P2 covers present four vocational preferences, overall vocational goals both short and long term. P3 is the plan for the current goal with 3 columns given to specific objectives, strategies and person/s responsible. P4 is the signing off point for both client and EC.
	10. **Review of Individual Employment Plan** A review of the IEP that may be followed by a new IEP.

expressed in a series of forms that are used to frame the relationship between the service and its clients. Protocols #1, 2, 3, 4, 7 and 8 do different things but they share in common their contribution to ensuring that the client's relationship to the service is one of informed consent. Protocols #5, 6, 7, 8, 9 and 10 all contribute to shaping a strategic partnership between the client and the service (worker) that manages the process of seeking and keeping employment for the individual client. Protocols #5, 6, 7, 8, 9 and 10 are also critical to ensuring that the service is individualized in the sense of being designed around the wants and needs of a particular client. They ensure that the service is client-centred. We examine the relationship between the forms and the living reality of the service delivery relationship in the next section.

We now situate these protocols as they are used in this service. The adoption of this approach requires a commitment from service workers to interweave the filling out of forms with the building of a dialogical and mutually accountable relationship with their clients. For this kind of commitment to be possible, a number of conditions have to be obtained. The service has to be free enough from government control and direction to be able to design and practise client-centred service provision. The workers have to be trained and supported in using these protocols creatively and flexibly in relation to the changing needs and wants of individuals. And the clients have to be sufficiently free of duress of various kinds to be able to creatively use the service and what it offers. Finally, the type and level of funding has to be of a kind that permits the service to do what its clientele needs it to do.

Our case study involves a service that was still block-funded by government (a regime that was changing by the end of our fieldwork). Also it represented a service type that was new, and this particular service, being one of the pioneers of this service type, had enjoyed considerable freedom in evolving the service protocols and quality standards that served its clientele. The clients were voluntary clients in the sense of 'choosing' to come to this service, a choice perhaps not so wide given the relatively few employment services that specialize in psychiatric disability. More significantly, at the time of study, if they were recipients of public income support, most likely the Disability Support Pension, they did not feel much pressure from government to become employed, and in this sense their decision to pursue employment was genuinely their own. This factor was also changing by the time of the end of our fieldwork.

The features of contract in service delivery

Table 12.2 presents the 11 features of contract in service delivery that we think are important. We have derived them both from our own work and from some of the literature on contract in social work (Maluccio and Marlow 1974; Seabury 1976). We discuss each feature in turn.

Table 12.2   The features of contract in individualized service delivery

---

- Differential participation of worker and client
- Mutual agreement
- Reciprocal accountability
- Explicitness
- Realism
- Flexibility
- Individualized strategic planning (management by objectives)
- Documentation (a paper trail of contractual nodes of the relationship)
- Structure for task, process, relationship, review and evaluation
- Informed consent
- Contractualized process of stages to the relationship (entry, establishment, intensive delivery, phasing out or maintenance, termination)

In our interviews with both workers and clients in our service case study no one was drawn to the language of contract as a way of capturing what they think to be good and valuable about this service and its service delivery relationship.[4] However, they do put emphasis on agreement, a sense of mutual responsibility and ownership, as well as on the kind of flexibility that promotes service individualization.

We begin with the relationship between worker and client because this has a foundational status with regard to all the other features of individualized service delivery. The features implicate each other and in this sense they accumulate as distinct aspects of what might be termed a contractualist approach to service delivery.

The *first* feature of contractualist service delivery is a term we take from Maluccio and Marlow (1974): *differential participation*, referring to the fact that the client and worker are engaged in a division of labour that positions them as different kinds of participant in their relationship. It is because they have different roles in the relationship that they both can and are required to collaborate for it to be an effective and successful relationship.

The worker's role is defined in terms of facilitating the client's pursuit of his/her own goals. The client's role is to assume responsibility for the pursuit of his/her own goals with facilitation and help. The boundaries of their respective roles and of their collaboration follow from these definitions. So also does the asymmetry in their respective power in the relationship, a difference in power that the worker (and the service agency that manages the worker) can use either to further the facilitation of client individuation or to hinder it.

Just whether and how contract is used in differential participation is the key to the individualization of service delivery. If contract is used by the worker just as a form to be signed off on rather than providing an ethical orientation and process for the relationship then a serious engagement of the client in the process of service delivery is not likely to occur.

The division of labour between worker and client, and its mediation by contract, are built into the *Vocational Profile* stage of the assessment process. Discussion with the client of all the issues in getting this form filled in gives the worker a good idea of where the individual is at in terms of vocational goals, established skills, confidence level, and understanding of how his/her illness may affect his/her employment. The same process offers a framework for dialogue between worker and client about both this individual's goals and what each needs to do for them to be achieved. It becomes obvious from how a worker, Robyn, talks about the process that the forms provide structure and prompts for a delicate process of communicative interaction between worker and client.[5] In this way, the forms provide the anatomy for a living entity, the relationship that is developing between the two:

> So we start with the general [question] if you could work anywhere what would you like to do, what would you like to be. Some people have trouble with this, they just cannot imagine beyond what they have done ... well no what do you want to be? We [also] get [the] donkey stuff, what geographical area do you want to work in, how far are you willing to travel, what conditions in the job are important to you? And then we look at what are you [the client] doing? Already he [Philip whose file we were examining with the worker] was already starting to look through the employment sections in papers himself, he was keeping his skills up to date. He wanted to get his presentation skills up, maintain his mental health in a positive way. And that five years time one which is always hard to answer; he wanted to have some responsibility, be financially secure, thought of as part of a team. We get a little bit into what kind of, how do you think your life will change once you start working so we can get a bit of an idea of where people are at, what are [the things] we are going to have to think about. Getting people to talk about their own qualities

is useful as well I find. Philip had a strong work history and had a lot of skills, he had a lot of stuff to work with. He saw himself with a lot of personal qualities. This was good for Philip to do this bit actually.

Philip's interviews with us indicate something of the importance to him of this process as well as both its delicacy and complexity:

They [the service] gave me my self-confidence back. [Question: And how did they do that?] Well they dwelt on the things that I could do ... Look at this, rather than saying that I failed at this or I failed at that, or I couldn't, look at what you can do. Let's write it down, lets have a list and I started to see things and their belief in me.

Later in the same interview on being asked 'what was it like to be asked questions about what is your goal, your aim?' Philip said:

Well that was confronting because I had to sit back and look. I must admit I had drifted a certain extent since I left the [military] ... I grew up thinking I was going to be in the [military].

In our second interview with Philip he spoke of the belief the service agency workers had in their clients, and brought out the collaborative nature of the relationship between worker and client:

Those people believe in you. They aren't just doing a job. Or if they are, they're doing a damn good [job] ... But they believe in their clients ... For me the worst part about mental health is not being able to trust yourself. ... And you're very alone because you can't trust yourself. You feel very helpless. And then, someone comes along who believes in you and you start to think, 'hang-on, I can do that'. And you're taken through little steps, like I said, very subtle ... I was very much involved. It wasn't somebody running my case, it was the two of us sorting it through together and that really happened. That was tremendous. It really was.

Disclosure of having a socially stigmatized type of illness to employers is a major issue for this client group. Discussion between worker and client on this issue is critical for determining whether and when to disclose in the process of job search. In the *Agreed Disclosure Authority* form the client indicates against each of the positions s/he has identified as ones s/he would like to try for whether s/he wants to disclose his/her mental illness to the employer. The worker is bound by the client's wishes on this matter. They also guide how the worker approaches an employer since obviously the worker cannot provide upfront employment support if a client has not disclosed. The *Ongoing Health Strategy* form is an instrument for provoking discussion and thought, about warning signs the client needs to be aware of for recurrence of his/her illness. Robyn's comments are suggestive of the significance of this transaction and bring out how a contractualist protocol mediates the differential participation *and* power of worker and client:

> If and when things go off the rails and preparing people [for this] ... Being aware of it rather than having that bandaid approach of when something does go wrong and suddenly trying to work out how to save that person's job or get them the help that they need ... It's not an easy form to get people to do because I have had people get upset because you are assuming they're going to get unwell again and they say but I'm not going to get unwell again. There is a bit of art in selling these forms. But it is a useful thing.

The *second* feature of contractualist service delivery, *mutual agreement* (see Maluccio and Marlow 1974) refers to the importance of the worker and the client negotiating and agreeing upon the nature and goals of their interaction and how they will proceed to meet those goals. This means emphasis on the worker following the client's own goals and facilitating processes by which the client comes to discover his/her own goals. Such an emphasis is likely to be evident in services oriented to adults who need intensive support for the acquisition of new skills and capabilities. However, if a worker finds that an individual is unsocialized, for example in what a prospective employer expects of punctuality and work dress, then the worker has to become more directive of the client. Such direction is however located within the agreement both worker and client share as to what it is they are trying to achieve and how from the standpoint of the advancement of the client's needs and wants.[6]

The *third* feature of contract in individualized service delivery is *reciprocal accountability*. It refers to the fact that 'the client and the worker are accountable to each other in various ways, each having an ongoing responsibility to fulfil agreed upon tasks and work toward agreed-upon goals' (Maluccio and Marlow 1974, 32). The specification of who has agreed to do what and by when is written down, and signed off by both parties, as in the *Individual Employment Plan* (IEP) type of contract. In this protocol, the client's current goal frames the top of the page of the form, after which follows a table of three columns: respectively, 'specific objectives', 'strategies', 'person/s responsible'. Marie was another client who gave us permission to access and use her file. Marie is in a maintenance phase of relationship to the service. She sees her worker on a weekly basis for ongoing support. In her most recent IEP (to which we had access), her current goal was 'maintain position at [employer] and increase value within organisation'. A specific objective was 'maintain good health' in relation to which she listed strategies that included:

- see doctor on a regular basis
- maintain regular sleeping patterns
- take medication daily
- ensure that anxieties are verbalized with Kate [her worker].

In this case 'person/s responsible' was Marie against each of these lines except for line four where it is Kate and Marie who are identified as responsible.

This degree of formalization permits easy review of whether in fact each has carried out their agreed upon course of action, and of whether and how it has furthered the goals of the client. Such review thus permits any rethinking of client readiness for such action or of the goals themselves that seems to be indicated by what has happened or not happened to date.

The contract remains client-centred, that is, focused on and driven by the client's goals as these are legitimized and supported by the worker operating within the mission and objectives of the service agency. These are not contracts designed to produce or compel compliance. If a client does not do what they undertook to do, this failure is not registered as a breach of contract that requires some kind of disciplinary sanction. Rather, the worker engages the client in asking why it is s/he did not do as s/he had agreed, what stopped them, or made it difficult for them to do this. This will reveal issues that have to be dealt with if the client is to be able to continue. For instance in the disability specialist employment service we have looked at, it is often the case that clients who have been mentally ill have either lost or never acquired life planning skills that are central to the whole cycle of getting up on time to get to work, have fresh clothes to wear, and maintain an adequate level of diet to sustain them. The worker's presumption in the case of client failure to do what they undertook to do will be either that they lack the skills and knowledge to do this, or, that maybe they are becoming ill again. In effect, there is no sanction for client failure to undertake what s/he agreed to do. In the event of sustained unwillingness or inability to meet their responsibilities, the service would terminate the client's relationship to it. Such termination follows from the reciprocal agreement that structures the client's entry to the service where the service specifies what it can offer and what it expects from the client.

In turn, the worker is accountable for what it is s/he has agreed to do in relation to a client. In the service we have examined there are several points at which the accountability of the worker gets called. Firstly, within the Individual Employment Plans which specify what the worker and the client will each do, when these plans are reviewed, the attention is on what each has agreed to do and whether it has been done. Secondly, the right to complain and how to use it is explained in the *Service Information Handbook* and this section comes after another full-page section on service user rights. Thirdly, the service oversights the worker's interaction with the client through periodic audit of the agreements that have been co-signed by the worker and client (see Table 12.1 above). This audit is in line with the quality assurance procedures of the service, and these have been designed to umbrella the service contractualist protocols we are discussing.

The *fourth* feature is *explicitness*. Maluccio and Marlow (1974, 33) usefully define this as 'the quality of being specific, clear, and open'. They (1974, 33) proceed to say:

> The contract offers an opportunity to spell out as openly as possible the conditions, expectations, and responsibilities inherent in the planned interaction ... To the traditional [social work] exhortation to 'start where the client is' might be added: 'and let him know where you are, and where you are going'. An explicit contract can help give the client more ethical protection than is possible through unspoken or covert contracts.

It is not just the worker that is required to be explicit. So too is the client. Maluccio and Marlow (1974, 33) suggest this is important because explicit 'contract formulation would actively engage the client's cognitive functions and resources—and such engagement has proved valuable in crisis intervention'. A good example in the case we are considering is the *Ongoing Health Strategy*. In this form the client is asked to name his/her warning signs of recurrent illness after being cued in on this question by a section which starts:

> Each person has their own pattern of warning signs, which usually occur just before an episode ... It is important to recognise your warning signs as they tend to be similar each time. For some people their warning signs may be triggered by stress, such as a major family crisis or starting work for the first time, after a long break.

This section is followed by another 'lead' or 'prompt' section which is titled 'What can I do when warning signs occur?', and which says 'it is important to have a plan of action worked out before warning signs appear' so that the client gets the treatment and support s/he needs. So the client is not asked just to fill out what their warning signs are but also to fill out a list of actions that respond to the question 'When I notice any of the warning signs I will: (a), (b), (c), (d).'

The *fifth* feature of contract in service delivery is *individualized strategic planning* or management by objectives (see Shaddock and Bramston 1991). The client and worker explicitly agree on what are to be the objectives for the client to work to meet, what strategies will be adopted to meet those objectives, and who will do what. This is the structure of the individual employment planning process. The plan is a rolling strategic plan, one that is subject to ongoing review and modification in the light of the client's achievements, changes of mind, or of condition, and experiences. In the case of Marie's individual employment planning referred to above, her current IEP supersedes her previous one in her file (which is stamped 'superseded').

The *sixth* feature of contract for individualized service delivery is *realism* (see Seabury 1976, 17). It is important that both client and worker set realistic goals. In our case study this includes the client learning a new level of management of his/her illness in relation to what it means to seek and keep employment. It is important also that the worker is realistic about what s/he can do or not do for the client, both in terms of resources available and the boundaries of his/her role as an employment consultant. On the latter front workers reported some difficulties in our interviews with them partly because there is a 'grey area' lying between employment support and life support,[7] and partly because the mental health specialist back-up was not always available, a fact these workers attributed to cut-backs in community mental health services.

The *seventh* feature of contract in service delivery is *flexibility*, that is the 'contract' is driven and shaped by the living and developing reality of the contractualized relationship between individual client and worker where there is ongoing adjustment and review of what is being aimed for and how. Seabury (1976, 17) says that this kind of contract 'is dynamic and flexible':

> Unlike legal contracts which by their very nature are designed to be static and binding, a social work contract can be renegotiated whenever a client or worker thinks that the terms are unfair and nonproductive or that they fail to include some important aspect of the social work process. Social work contracts are not written to be *a priori* rules to cover all contingencies nor are they expected to be followed blindly.

The *eighth* feature of contract is *documentation, the paper trail* that the various contractualist documents constitute. Thus they can be subject not only to review by the service team of client and worker but to the review and audit of third parties, including service management. In the recurrent possibility of a worker moving on, or a client changing his/her worker, there is a paper trail to be consulted by the new worker for the client. In the service we studied, this paper trail was carefully maintained as an individual client's file but it was not a routine practice for the service to give clients a copy of the forms/agreements they had signed off on with their worker. Marie's worker Kate gave her a copy of her IEP, and Marie was the kind of client who would have wanted her own written copy to consider and consult. Marie before she became ill was a skilled and experienced personal assistant who worked in a prestigious international agency. By occupation as well as by the reflexive demands of coming to terms with being mentally ill in her middle age, she is likely to see such a paper trail as important. Marie told us:

> I think it's better to have it written down because you can refer back to it and that's what we do. Every six months we review the previous one. And often, it doesn't change too much. You know, for

the forthcoming period. But, it's a good discipline for me to have some guidelines, that it provides.

We consider that if the paper trail is to work for both client and worker, and to remain client-centred, then it is important for clients to have their own copies.

Not all clients value the paper trail although our data suggests that most regard the formal IEP process as useful in retrospect even if at the time they were confused about its significance. The workers also divided into those who saw the paper trail and its demands as a necessary evil, and those who valued it highly. Kate was one of the latter. On being asked in our interview with her what she found good and useful or not good and useful about the individual employment plan process, she answered:

> I don't find anything not good about them. I think they're excellent tools to first of all keep focused with a client, when you meet with them on a regular basis to sort of refer back to the employment plan, refer back to what the agreed strategies are. It's a good objective piece of negotiation that we can refer to. I think they're also good because if a client has a particular goal, we can cut that goal up into however many little pieces there needs to be. So the client can see that they are moving towards achieving their goals.

The *ninth* feature of contract is implicit in the others, namely that contract is a means of providing *structure for the task, process of interaction and the relationship* that are involved in service provision. This structure is formalized to the extent that it is named and made explicit in conformity with written service protocols, service standards and guidelines.

The *tenth* feature of contract, that is especially important in our case, is *informed consent*. The client is not asked to sign off on anything without being informed appropriately about what is involved and without general information about his/her rights, including especially the right to confidentiality and privacy.

The *eleventh* feature of contract in service provision is that it is a *contractualist process of distinct stages* in the negotiation of the service relationship from point of referral to termination. Seabury (1976, 17) identifies five stages: (1) *exploration and negotiation* which covers the referral, entry and assessment stages in this service; (2) the *preliminary contract* stage which covers the transition from assessment into the negotiation of the first IEP in this service; (3) *the working contract* which covers the IEP, its review, and the development of further IEPS and their review; (4) *phasing out or maintenance* which covers ongoing low-key support to clients who have been successful in gaining and keeping employment; and (5) *termination*, when a client no longer needs/wants such ongoing support or when the service decides it cannot assist a client because after a considerable period of time checking out their readiness for employment, it is clear that no progress is being made.

The limits of contract in service delivery

Contract is central to the democratization of the service delivery relationship, but its use must be embedded within the living relationship between the service (worker) and the client. Contracts will be only as good as they are used, so the emphasis should be on contracts in use, on staff training to use them, and on the values by which they are to be oriented.

The use of contract may lead to an implicit 'creaming', i.e. preference for clients who are cognitively, lingually, and culturally comfortable with a contractualist process. In our case study, we noted that the clients and workers who liked and valued the contractualist aspect were people who were not just educated but inclined to self-reflection. Thus contract may be good for people who are drawn to what Giddens (1991) calls strategic life planning but less useful to people whose relationship to life is more tacit, intuitive, and perhaps less obsessive-compulsive.

Thirdly, most contracts we know of tend to be service-led and -oriented in their design but there is no inherent necessity for this. If contracts are to facilitate the democratization of client status, client advocates and representatives need to be involved in discussion about the use and design of contract in democratic service delivery. Carnaby (1997) and Shaddock and Bramston (1991) suggest that individual planning processes for people with learning disabilities tend to be professionally driven, with relatively low involvement of clients in the process. Carnaby (1997, 382) comments of services in Britain that they 'still concentrate on the outcomes of individual planning rather than the nature of user involvement and the meaning that the service holds for the user'.

Fourthly, contract in service delivery is good for voluntary clients, namely in service settings where the relatively greater power of the service worker in relation to the client generally does not involve the use of force. Contract can and should be used with involuntary clients, but it can also be more easily abused. Abuse of contract occurs when contract is used not to structure the participation of the client in the process but to force pseudo-consent to an imposed process. Seabury's (1976, 19) comments of involuntary clients that the problem 'is how to establish a mutual agreement or a common ground when the client fails to recognise a problem or does not look on the worker as someone who can be of service'. He adds: 'Many of the techniques of working with this client population boil down to persistence and a highly client-centred focus.' The question of how contract can be used with individuals who have been mandated into treatment—as in the increasing use of legal tools 'to mandate treatment adherence in the community' (Monahan *et al.* 2001, 1198; and see also Campbell *et al.* 2006) for people with mental illness—is an important question (see note 1). In principle, publicly accountable and constitutionally regulated use of coercion can be reconciled with procedural justice; and it may be reasonable to impose expectations of treatment regime compliance on people if they are receiving a genuine service. That said there are clearly more and less rights-oriented models of mandated or community treatment orders available at this time and the former should not be confused with the latter.[8] Moreover, as Monahan *et al.* 2001, 1202, comment, 'it is not yet clear that services that are effective when received voluntarily produce the same outcomes when they are received under duress'.

Government and the democratization of service delivery

We have used a case study in order to help us think about what role contractualism can play in democratizing the service delivery relationship. If the autonomy of individual clients is to be respected, and service is to be individualized, the service delivery relationship is the critical point of policy implementation.

Our case is that of a service that crafted a contractualist approach to service delivery. Towards the end of our fieldwork period, it was clear that government policy was changing the conditions of operation for this service, and that it would be forced to shift from a block grant to case-based funding. The funding will now be attached to 'cases', and the total amount allocated to each case will be allocated in proportions at key points of the case moving through the service and into employment. In fact, there are funding caps attached to different categories of client located on a scale of need for more to less intensive assistance.

By requiring the service to treat everyone the same way in a standardized set of time lines for the process of assessment, job search and successful employment placement, its capacity to offer a genuinely individualized service is likely to be reduced. Case-based funding, like most quasi market funding regimes, makes no provision for the infrastructural (e.g. staff training and service development) costs of service delivery. In this respect, it is to be contrasted with competitive tendering funding regimes where a provider can submit a price that reflects the real costs of delivering the service.[9]

The point of service delivery *is* the critical level at which the democratization and individualization of service delivery can occur, but only if government policy and funding positively frame and support service delivery so conceived. Service deliverers who have achieved best practice in the democratization of the service delivery relationship have much to offer to discussions of policy and program management. The question of the conduct of the service delivery relationship is a question of its governance. It is important that democratic and constitutionalist thinking be brought to bear on the conduct of the service delivery relationship and on how it is framed by the wider work of government.

Notes

1 In response to the first version of this chapter (published as a journal article) we have been advised that ours is the only paper that applies relational contract theory to services for people with mental illness by a US-based researcher working with the MacArthur Foundation on the topic of mandated community treatment, John Petrilo, Department of Mental Health Law & Policy, University of South Florida. In email communication to Anna Yeatman (9 April 2007) he says that one of the questions his research network is considering is 'what legal principles might provide an adequate framework for considering long-term relationships in which a person is required to participate in treatment'. This is clearly an important question to work on.

2 This service does not provide supervision for its workers even though there is a 'clinical' aspect of their work with people who have a mental illness.

3 The service is paying award rates, and is doing what it can to top them up by providing each worker with a car as well as 3% penalty rates.

4 Two of the employment counsellors distinguished between how they work with clients in this service and how contract gets used to structure and even force compliance in mental health settings. Richard's comment is generally representative of staff feeling on the matter: 'There's an informal contract. I don't know what the clients would think of that. Whether they'd even think that there was some sort of contract. It's more of an agreement or an arrangement of working together. It seems too hard, contract.'

5   This is an edited part of a transcript of a long discussion we had with Robyn as she took us through Philip's file where all the signed-off contractualist protocols we were interested in were kept. We did not get this access to this file until after we had interviewed the client concerned, and had obtained his consent to look at his file with his employment consultant, the worker. After which we obtained his consent to copy his file so that we were able to refer to it as a source of data.

6   The worker is likely to direct the client when it is an issue of client needs as discerned by the worker, and when his/her wants are not adequately in line with his needs. A client needs to be punctual in turning up to his/her employment on time. The role of the workers is to bring the client to an understanding that the pursuit of his/her desire for employment entails this need, and thus bringing his/her wants in line with his/her needs. Such direction might be termed contractualist paternalism and is not necessarily at odds with respect for the client's agency (see Clark 1998).

7   On this Kate's remarks in her interview with us are instructive: 'Where does your role stop and start? At what point are we entering into a territory that perhaps his case manager or psychologist or whatever is dealing with. It's very grey. Again you know you might have someone who has schizophrenia and their main barrier might be that they get really paranoid, or they get, they feel like people are talking about them. They might even hear voices. They might think the co-workers are talking about them. So that might be the main barrier to them keeping a job. So therefore, in an employment plan, you should be addressing these issues if that's what they're for. But again, what's the difference between that and a plan that a case manager or a mental health team would be writing? It's grey.'

8   For an interesting 'rights-oriented' model see the discussion of Community Treatment Orders in Ontario by Campbell *et al.* 2006, 1107–1108.

9   For a results-oriented funding system that does work with the real costs of service provision and that has been designed and implemented by means of a three-way stakeholder partnership involving the funding government agency, providers, and consumers, see the Oklahoma model as described by its developer, Dan O'Brien with others, see Novak *et al.* (1999).

13
Are Prisoners Clients? The Individualization of Public Correctional Services

Diane Gursansky and Anna Yeatman

> *Well we had this dream that a person would go to prison, they would be assessed, a plan would be prepared for them and that the time in the system, whether it be in lock up or on release, would follow the plan. ... And that it would end up connecting them to their going back into the world and that they would ... have more skills, and they would have had their issues dealt with to some extent. And their families would have been involved in that too. That was the simple vision. It is not a silly vision. It is a thing that ... drives you to ask what do you have to do to make this happen* (from interview with Sue Vardon 2001).

Introduction

Prisoners as clients, how could this be so? Prisoners are criminals, offenders, society's reprobates, sometimes monsters and always guilty! Clients are people seeking help, paying for expertise, negotiating for a service they want, and they are customers so far as they are able to voice dissatisfaction with a service, perhaps even to exit this service agency in order to find another one more to their liking. This is the sense in which Patrick Weller (1997) understands the term and idea of 'client': prisoners are not clients for whatever they are their situation is neither voluntary nor do they have a choice of which corrections agency that they are to be located within.

The language of client belongs within a professional service. The fact of being positioned in an involuntary relationship to a human service does not disqualify the individual from being considered a client of this service. As Sue Vardon (1997, 127) points out in her exchange with Weller on the question of whether prisoners should be considered clients, 'the concept of the involuntary client is very familiar to those people working in statutory agencies—the social work literature has explored this'. Vardon (1997, 127) goes onto to say: 'Those working in child protection, community corrections and juvenile justice rely on ... [this concept] for the development of their philosophical and theoretical models for intervention'. Vardon's reasoning is informed by the service ethic of professions like social work, generic human services, law, health and psychology, and she assumes that these professions both should and do shape the statutory institutional worlds of involuntary clients.

Weller (1997, 126) agrees that prisoners receive services within prison: 'food, clothing, medical services, educational counselling and training; all that is required to allow them to live securely and safely for the period for which they have been sentenced and to have the opportunity for rehabilitation'. He agrees also that the prison has to be viewed, at least in part, as an environment of service provision to prisoners. However, the fact that prisoners are not voluntary clients, are subject to discipline, and are chronically dissatisfied with their lot (Weller 1997, 126) for Weller means that it makes no sense to view them as clients, let alone as customers!

Historically in prisons, the language used has been one that creates a special identity for the person who is in prison that sets him or her aside from the mainstream of welfare service clients: offender, prisoner, inmate or remandee. The term client may be used by specialist professional staff (e.g. lawyers, psychologists or social workers) but it would not be the term used by prison officers and managers. While from the 1970s onwards, the rhetoric of prisoner rights and the movement of deinstitutionalization impacted on prisons,[1] the custodial aspect of correctional services has prevailed until recently. Prisons have been the only continuing legitimate expression of the old institutional order of warehousing people that has otherwise disappeared, or at least in the case of orphanages, insane asylums, and institutional warehouses for children with developmental disabilities, become discredited.

Yet, over the last couple of decades, the world of correctional services has been integrated into the new service and outcomes-oriented emphases of the new public management (NPM). While there has been a longstanding tension between liberal-rehabilitative and security/control approaches to the management of prisoners inside prisons (Liebling 2003), currently there is a rethinking of both these approaches in relation to managing prisoners as both instantiations of a category *and* as individuals, better. The two approaches converge in the idea of combining a societal interest in reducing re-offending with the individual prisoner's interest in having options other than re-offending open to him or her in the conduct of his or her life. The prisoner's interest is identified with services that are oriented to the enhancement of his or her functioning (Ward and Stewart 2003). It is a rehabilitative approach that assumes that a criminal repertoire of behaviour reflects 'compromised and impaired' individual functioning that has come about because the individual has faced major obstacles to the meeting of their basic needs for autonomy, relatedness and competence, and have resorted to 'adopt defensive strategies and substitute or "proxy" needs' (Ward and Stewart 2003, 138).

This chapter focuses on the introduction of an individualized service approach to the management of prisoners in South Australia in the period 1993–1997. This is discussed in context of contemporary trends in prison management both internationally and in Australia. The case study is based in data collected by Diane Gursansky which comprise: an interview undertaken in 2001 with Sue Vardon who had been the chief executive officer of the South Australian Department of Correctional Services in the period 1994–1997; Departmental *Annual Reports* from 1994–1995 through to 1998/1999; access to presentations by South Australian Correctional Services management to the Case Management Society of Australian Conference in 2000; and an evaluation of the first stages of implementing case management in South Australian prisons by social work students under the supervision of Diane Gursansky in her role as a social work academic/educator in the Unisversity of South Australia. The South Australian data have been supplemented with data gathered by Anna Yeatman from an interview with Luke Grant of the New South Wales Department of Corrective Services in 2003 in order to assess common trends and the culture of understanding amongst senior managers in the world of Australian correctional services.

Three themes stand out in relation to this case study. Firstly, the new conception of individualizing welfare services 'mainstreams' one of the most stigmatized groups in society—convicted offenders—and brings them into the category of individuals who are service clients or customers. They become thought of as individuals who deserve respect, whose conduct as offenders is intelligible because it reflects their life experience and the subjective sense they have made of it, and who therefore belong within rather than outside the world of human services. Ward and Marshall (2007, 279) refer to this non-stigmatizing approach to offenders in terms of the idea of 'narrative identity': 'There is characteristically a purpose, a logic in what offenders do and why they do it.'[2]

Secondly, the new public management emphasis on outcomes is one that can have an individualizing impetus. The conception of outcomes is tied to change in what it is that people as individuals are able to be and do, change that can be facilitated and supported by appropriate service interventions. Just warehousing or parking people is not acceptable; instead there has to be measurable results, in this case the reduction of re-offending by convicted offenders. This outcome cannot be achieved without designing corrections as an effective service intervention which assists convicted offenders as individuals in changing whatever it is they need to change in their skills and conduct in order not to re-offend. The new thinking of offenders as individuals and 'whole persons' is not simply driven by the value of respect but by consideration of how they are individuals whose action reflects their experience of the world and the options it offers them. If they are to change, then they have to acquire new subjective experience that makes new behavioural options meaningful. Certainly, there is a fundamental ambiguity built into the designated outcome in this service arena: in aiming to reduce re-offending, is the focus on the prisoner's interest, on that of the wider community, or on both? The current rhetoric of Correctional Services emphasize compatibility between these two interests.

Thirdly, case management is the key service technology in the adaptation of the whole corrections system to an individualized service approach, with individualized treatment plans becoming the *modus operandi* for clinical (psychological and social work) intervention in relation to individual offenders (for a human-rights oriented conception of correctional clinical practice see Ward and Birgden 2007). Key to the introduction of case management in the correctional system is the introduction of an electronic individual client file that supplies a continuous and updated base of information including, most likely, a risk assessment profile of the individual (assessment geared to the likelihood of re-offending) and the results of treatment intervention. The importance of an electronically managed file that follows the individual across the different system components in this service arena is an interesting point of comparison with another group that is also highly vulnerable to system neglect and abuse, children in out of home care, as discussed in Chapter 9.

International trends in contemporary prison management

Issues of prison management and the treatment of offenders have attracted a significant literature over the last couple of decades primarily because of the increasing use of incarceration as punishment for serious and repeat offenders over the last 20 years (see for example, Beck 1999; Carlson and Garrett 1999; Lauen 1997; Hass and Alpert 1998; Welch 1996; Crow 2001). In commenting on the situation in the USA, Beck (1999, 44), Welch (1996, 124) and Lauen (1997, 5) argue that during the 1980s and 1990s the get-tough policies have seen a tripling in the number of adults under some form of correctional supervision. These policies have resulted in higher arrest rates, dramatic increase in drug law violations, more first term offenders, tougher sentencing and increased severity of prison terms. While the USA has led the way in higher incarceration rates, similar trends are evident internationally. For prison managers the challenge has been to contain costs, minimize violence in overcrowded prisons, meet political and community expectations of tough responses to convicted offenders, while yet ensuring reduction in re-offending or recidivism (Stojkovic and Farkas 2003; Lauen 1997).

New thinking about prison management has advocated a more individualized approach to the management of prison populations (Hass and Alpert 1998, 350–351). Two new strategies emerged in the USA from the 1970s: first, unit management and, then, case management. Carlson and Garrett (1999, 85) and Houston (1999, 322) describe *unit management* as the decentralization of prison management where a large prison is broken up into smaller units of prisoner management with the same group of prison officers assigned to work with the same group of individual prisoners over time. Where it is possible to design new prisons for unit management, this of course has assisted this new initiative. These writers identify the strengths of the unit management with decisions about inmates that are made by staff who know them best, and with the improvement of relationships between prisoners and staff thereby reducing incidents of violence and leading to improved morale of prisoners and staff. Under these conditions it is argued that greater efficiency is achieved across the three functions of prisons: correction, care and control of the prisoner (Carlson 1999, 85–86; Houston 1999, 325). *Case management* is designed to focus service on the needs of the prisoner as an individual, to approach them as a 'whole person' whose progress through the corrections system from entry to exit needs tracking by means of an accessible and continuous individual client file that informs the case plan adopted for this individual. The key element of case management in prisons is a case plan that is designed in relation to each individual offender's profile and an evidence-based assessment of the risk of his/her re-offending. The goals are to provide an individualized approach to service based on comprehensive assessment/classification of the individual from the point of admission into the system through to the transition back to the community (Carlson 1999, 83–85) and to integrate prisons and community corrections into a single service system that is oriented to the effective management of individual offenders.

The Australian scene

Similar trends and issues to those reported above are evident in Australia. Brown and Wilkie (2002, xxiv) comment that the most significant feature of the Australian context is an escalating prison population, both in absolute numbers and as a proportion of the general population. This trend reflects higher arrest rates, increasing use of mandatory sentencing, longer sentencing and 'truth in sentencing' policies (Dawes 2002, 114). Hogg (2002, 5) states that in 18 years the daily prison rate has increased by almost two-thirds and expenditure on justice increased 23%: 'As a consequence of these trends over the last two decades present imprisonment rates are higher than they have been at any time since the beginning of the twentieth century (Hogg 2002, 4)'.

Dawes (2002, 114) discusses the 1970s as a period when governments advanced prisoners rights within an era of administrative reform (see Yeatman 1990 Chapter 1; Wilenski 1986, Chapter 9). In the 1980s when managerialism displaced administrative reform, the value of efficiency often threatened to crowd out the value of equity (see Wilenski 1986, Chapter 2) but there was a continuous emphasis on customizing service to need (both as objectively imputed and subjectively expressed). The correctional services system was not exempt from these reform agendas. By the 1990s as governments began to use law and order rhetoric to court electorates, and introduced a more punitive approach to offenders, the new public management emphasis on a cost effective service that achieved the result of reducing re-offending prevailed. The refraction of a populist rhetoric of law and order through a public management emphasis on the efficient achievement of positive results created a window of opportunity for the adoption of an individualized service approach to offenders.

Over the last 20 years, like their overseas counterparts, Australian prisons have introduced new strategies of prison management. Although the rate of change has varied from state to state, the introduction of unit management and later case management has been a consistent trend. Unit management was well in place in the 1980s and case management was increasingly adopted during the 1990s. The first states to introduce case management were New South Wales (Feenan 2000),

Victoria, Queensland and South Australia (ICAC 1998; McBride 2000). At the present time all other states and territories have moved to case management.

The recent reform of South Australian Correctional Services

The agenda for change in South Australian prisons has conformed to the international and national trends. The last 20 years has seen a major refocusing of the task of prison management in response to the increasing size of prison populations, the challenges of maintaining security with populations that are volatile and diverse and community demands for reduction in offending behaviour. The community and governments want prisoners to be punished but also want them to return to society as more law abiding citizens. The current 'branding' of the South Australian Department for Correctional Services is expressed as 'contributing to a safer community by providing offenders with opportunities to stop offending'.

The scene was set for major reform in South Australia in 1993 after a change of government. The new Liberal Party government came to power after a crisis of confidence in the economic management of the state associated with the previous Labor Government. The Liberal Party's election campaign focused on the Labor Government's economic mis-management, its failure to curb union demands and to create an efficient and effective public service. The incoming Minister of Corrections held firm views about weaknesses in prison management and the system's inability to contain prisoner violence, drug usage and prison costs. The 1980s had seen tensions between prison unions and Government in relation to work conditions and pay claims and the new Government was determined to establish that it, not the unions, ruled the prisons. John Dawes (2002, 123), a former CEO of Correctional Services in South Australia, argues that a pathological antipathy between Government, prison officers and other public servants had created a climate in which the new Government was determined to break the existing control of the prison system by custodial staff and to open the system to more competitive and market oriented strategies.

Sue Vardon who became the chief executive officer (CEO) of Correctional Services under the new minister was the Commissioner for Public Employment; before that she had been the CEO of the Department of Community Welfare. By convention she offered her resignation as Commissioner for Public Employment to the new Government and negotiated a transfer to CEO of a line agency. She was offered Correctional

Services, and she accepted the job (from the interview with Sue Vardon 2001). Sue Vardon served as CEO of Correctional Services from December 1993 until she resigned to take up the position of CEO of the newly created Commonwealth Government one-stop-shop public income support service agency, Centrelink, in 1997 (see Chapter 8). Sue Vardon is a social worker by training and, in the course of her public sector career she has become established as leading figure in Australian NPM approaches especially to service delivery. In being offered the position of CEO of Correctional Services, Vardon was positioned as the new broom that would sweep the old undesirable culture and practices away and bring this Department into a NPM approach. She was practiced in adapting her agenda for reform to the elected government's reform rhetoric. She was skilled in working the relationship between herself as the CEO of a government department and her Minister. Her previous experience as a highly effective manager of the Department of Community Welfare ensured that she would be a tough and skilled advocate of the Department of Correctional Services as a claimant on government policy and resources.

With Vardon, then, came a professional and experienced approach to Correctional Services as one among other human services. Her social work background equipped her to readily understand and pick up the new emphasis on the case management of prisoners; and her public management reform background primed her to adopt a generic management approach to correctional services rather than to see them as a unique kind of public service environment demanding a distinctive management approach. In this case, the reorganization was oriented to breaking down the silo of the prison itself and reintegrating it into a wider system of correctional services as these include both prisons and the community arm of corrections (home detention, probation, parole and community service) in its articulation with the justice system, prisoners' families, and other relevant agencies.

Vardon as a CEO had been formed within the era associated with de-institutionalization, the shift from institutional to community care policy in sectors such as youth work, ageing, mental health and disability. The vehicle of community care was, at this time, case management. In this service approach the case manager is expected to work with the client to tailor services based on assessment of need, implement a service plan that involves cooperation across a number of providers, maintain a point of contact and continuity for the client, monitor progress and ensure that there is an appropriate response to changing circumstances so that declared outcomes can be achieved. These are the core elements of case management (Gursansky, Harvey and Kennedy 2003, 18).

Vardon came with this set of dispositions, experience, and knowledge to the job of CEO of South Australian Correctional Services at a time when a new Government and Minister wanted to make a decisive and public break with past practice and culture of this Department. Being herself an innovator and change manager, there was congruence between her orientation to her new leadership challenge and the Minister's insistence on changing old, entrenched ways. She commented in interview with us: 'So we shared the same goals but for quite, quite different reasons and I realized fairly quickly on that if I didn't put the reasons on the table but the aspiration on the table, we could find common ground'. If she could persuade the Minister that her methods would reduce re-offending, make prison management more accountable to Government goals, and be in line with best international evidence-based practice, then she was likely to win the political space within which to go to work.

She took some time to 'find the problem' as she put it in interview. When she looked at what was going on with the practiced eye of someone who understood integrated and systematic approaches to service delivery, she discovered that there was no programmatic service focus in South Australian prisons. Here are her own words in responding to the question where did she get the idea of introducing a case management approach from?

> Where did I get it from? First I found the problem. ... there was no concept that the prisoner was a whole person ... it was about what have we got on, oh you can go and do woodwork if you like and you would be halfway through a course and you would be moved because there would be too many people in that prison and then there was no way you could finish that course because every prison had their own different thing, there was no concept of articulation of anything. ... So all these prisoners had little bits and pieces of this stuff, none of which was going to be any good whatsoever when they got out into the community. At the same time we had knowledge about the prisoners that was not passed on, the only knowledge that was passed on was [whether] they [were] dangerous or not. ... It was gossip, it was reputational.

She went on to emphasize this point by saying that information about an individual offender was not shared between the prison and community-correctional service arms of the organization, nor was there any systemic approach to building a continuous file that profiled each prisoner and to understanding why the prisoner as an individual had engaged in offending in the first place. Thus she 'found' the problem: '[the Department] was not prisoner-centric'. Here are her words again:

> ... if you really believed we were there to stop them re-offending, which I felt was really fairly fundamental, another one of the things I tried to engage the Minister on, you had to understand why they offended in the first place and try ... [to] address [that] so they wouldn't offend again. ... [T]here was no way that this was all together and so we developed the notion of a file following a person.

Once Vardon 'found the problem', she was able to recognize what could help her address it. At a correctional services conference in Brisbane, she heard a presentation by two Canadian psychologists on addressing the improvement of cognitive skills in prisoners, and she immediately 'went straight up to them and said I want to hire you' to come and work with South Australian Correctional Services. Her next step is revealing of her skill in making her agenda and that of the Minister's come together:

> Then I had to work [out] how to get them there. And that was really interesting as [the Minister] didn't want to spend a single cent, certainly not on prisoners. So what I said to him was, I worked out how he thought, and I said to him, do you know that the worst things that happens to prisoners is that they sit around doing nothing [and planning their next crime].

She organized for the two Canadian psychologists to talk with the Minister, he 'bought the deal', and the money (in interview she recalls it as a quarter of a million dollars) was allocated to this initiative. Later in the interview Vardon reiterates her view that the only thing worth measuring in assessing the performance of prisons is whether they stop re-offending which is not what prisons have done in the past:

> They measure escapes and things like that, they don't measure stopping re-offending. ... there is a feeling that you will take them off the streets for a short period of time and we will be safe because

they are off the streets. It's such an appalling notion because they come back out, and they come back out worse than when they went in. So there has to be a fundamental belief, which not everyone shares, that you have got to make society safer because of what happens on the inside. And it's only through case management that I believe that can happen. Oh, and a significant experience also in cognitive skills. ... you have to have both.

In interview, Vardon said that 'we started with the concept of a file' that would follow each individual offender as they moved through the system. As with children in out of home care (Chapter 9), the client group is one that is highly vulnerable to accumulative and compounded social problems (for example violent or abusive family relationships, and non-completion of schooling leading to difficulties with employability) and to societal stigma. Historically, the individuals in both groups have been at risk of system neglect and abuse, not least of which has been the lack of systematic process in tracking and profiling these individuals as they are moved across different service agencies and locations over what can be a relatively long period of time. Thus in both cases the essential though not sufficient component of individualizing service has been the creation of an individual client file.

Starting with the concept of a file went along with the piloting of the introduction of a case management method of service provision in two prisons (Adelaide Women's and Port Augusta). Vardon comments of the importance of getting the Information Technology people to design and build an electronic client file that this was 'fundamental to the whole exercise': 'Because once you built it into the IT system, you can't get rid of it. You can but it's hard'.

Further development of the change process built on overseas experience and knowledge and consultants were brought in to train staff for new practices. Vardon was clear that the new vision had to be explicit and that she had to put work into changing people. Her strategy in changing people had several aspects. First she built her own management team. She appointed all new prison managers, giving retirement packages to most of the old ones, sacking or moving others. She worked intensively with her team in leading and supporting them: 'it was easier for me to say we were going to do some of these things and they would look at me and they would say, "Sue you don't know how hard it is for us to do that", and I would say, "yes I know"'. She says of her leadership style in relation to working with the key people in making the change happen, a style that she refined and matured in her role as CEO of Centrelink:

Sue: [In leading the change] you just become single minded, you say this is the way we are going. But you actually have to have the vision, it doesn't just come [over] night, you have to build [it], it's quite scientific ... I think the world is driven by informed people and ideologues. And in prison there are a lot of ideologues. What I had to do was actually put the pieces together and make a conceptual whole, and then try and go back to the pieces.

Interviewer: But you keep saying that you also [have to] find the person who can make that happen where you want it to happen.

Sue: Yes, but you have to stand behind them and I don't think anyone has felt abandoned by me, unless they are hopeless and then I have told them, and they have gone. But they were always pushed further than they can go but they were always strongly supported behind.

Changing the culture of prisons was a key component of her change strategy. Language was a central issue and Vardon began by talking about prisoners as one of the customer groups of the Department. The shift for prisoner officers to think about crims as customers caused considerable controversy. Vardon realized fairly quickly that she had to both train and empower prison officers if they were to come inside the new vision. We turn to discussion of this issue in the next two sections.

Vardon did not work in a vacuum. She was able to presuppose not just the wider environment that legitimized her vision but more specifically she was able to build on a reform process already under way within South Australian Correctional Services. In the late 1980s the former CEO had sent community corrections staff to Europe to look at unit management and case management. Unit management had been already adopted in the prisons but case management stayed within the community corrections section of the Department. Here it was colonized by the social work tradition of case work, for the probation and parole personnel were all social workers, so it is arguable that case management did not arrive until Vardon's time as CEO of the Department.

The challenge of individualizing the service relationship between prison officers and prisoners

Prisoners present complex bundles of problems relating to addiction, attachment, social competence, violence, sexual violence, mental health, and cognitive skills. Prison populations reflect the characteristics of compounded disadvantage and marginalization. Unless there is a management system that supports a case management type relationship between prison officers and prisoners as well as appropriate training and supervision of prison officers in a 'case officer' role, an individualized service relationship between prison officers and prisoners is an insuperable challenge. Moreover, without a value-oriented focus on the prisoner as an individual or whole person, it makes no sense to attempt the kind of reform that is under discussion in this chapter. Sue Vardon (1997, 128) makes this point eloquently:

> The majority of offenders in prison are young, impulsive, unstructured in their thinking, self-oriented and prone to blame others for their circumstances. They have traditionally been mass managed— passing through the system without being confronted with their behaviour, and so failing to mature. Age eventually catches up with them and they slow down but not before they reoffend. Fortunately, there are now evaluated programs which when delivered can significantly affect this type of individual. And that is the important word, the individual. The effective correctional system now assesses individuals and develops a plan for each which includes confronting them with their offending behaviour and providing alternative solutions when they are faced with the type of circumstances which usually leads to conflict with the law.
>
> People in prison do have a choice about whether they participate in the opportunities or not. Surprisingly many do want to change and take the opportunities to learn these as an alternative to work and to be educated. ...
>
> This relatively new approach only works when the staff inside also participate in the belief they are contributing to stopping reoffending. It requires the type of attitude we would expect in any human service agency working with clients—an individual-centred focus, a respectful attitude, skilled interpersonal contact, confidentiality and modelling.

Vardon encountered a number of difficulties in bringing both prison officers and the specialist staff into this new approach and attitude. Historically, prison officers have been positioned as the custodial staff whose role is segregated from the specialist professionals who offer clinical services both inside prisons and the community arm of correctional services. The specialist staff who work in the prison (such as medical staff, social workers, psychologists, teachers and prison workshop staff) and other outsiders who enter the prison such as specialist service providers, volunteers, maintenance workers, are let off the hook—they do not have to engage in the custodial management of prisoners. All enter the prison under the condition they will maintain the rules and restrictions imposed on prisoners but with more flexibility than custodial staff. The specialist staff posed a challenge in their own right for they had their own custom and practice which did not involve them in working collaboratively with either the clients or the prison officers. They did not want to share the client's file with the officers and to include them in case conferencing. Thus getting both the specialist staff and prison officers to work together and to include the individual prisoner in a collaborative approach to his/her case management was a significant challenge.

With new service expectations of them that they contribute as case officers to the case management of individual prisoners, prison officers still have to play the custodial role. There is an inherent tension between the new 'clinical' service role and their continuing custodial role. At the same time prison officers are generally much less educated and trained than the specialist staff, a hierarchically marked difference that informs the division of labor between these two categories of worker in correctional services, the former getting to do the 'heavy lifting' control work, the latter getting to do the nice guy clinical work. This difference is not easily resolved. Even with the introduction of a certified training course for prison officers, they continue to be less professionally educated than the social workers for example in the community arm of correctional services. For this reason the prison officers were positioned as case workers under the supervision of the professionally trained staff as case managers or coordinators.

To a degree the prisoner officers are also imprisoned within the same environment as the prisoners. They do of course leave after their shift and have the opportunity to maintain their social networks. They have a job to do but it is one that also isolates them from the wider community. There are limits on their freedom to talk about their work because of privacy issues and organizational discretion. When incidents occur they are required to deal with violence or threats to safety and their responsibilities can place them at risk of injury. Until recently, they have not been required to have anything other than on the job training for their work. The emphasis has been on the physical containment of difficult (and predominantly male) offenders who have the capacity to harm themselves and others. Custodial staff are there to maintain security and getting too close to prisoners, too personally involved in their situations has traditionally been considered dangerous and inappropriate practice.

Finally, prison officers shared the same social background of many of the offenders. In a colloquial 'insider' way of talking in interview with her, Vardon classified the offenders into three groups: those who were one-off offenders, were deeply ashamed and who would work hard to 'get out as fast as they can'; second, 'the naughty boys', the kids that teachers used to expel, and who 'muck around', who are 'not necessarily bad but ... will do spontaneous acts of naughtiness because that is part of their personality'; and, third, 'the really "sickos" who do terrible crimes'. She said of the difference between someone who had offended, 'especially that middle group, the naughty boys, and the prison officers' that it 'was hardly any difference at all', a fact that made the relationship between prison officers and offenders all the more complex:

> Paper thin, in fact they often knew each other. But the prison officers, because they weren't very well educated, did all that classic stuff about becoming the guards, and they would be cruel, they would tease, they would taunt, and they were just disrespectful. For the [individual] prison officer to be respectful, they would have to do it quietly, you know, because that was seen as not done.

Overcoming barriers to the change process

Vardon identified a number of barriers to change. Firstly, the Minister and Government saw Correctional Services as a portfolio that spelt trouble and this could lead the political level of the change process to be cynical about the possibilities of change and to seek solutions based in control not partnership. Secondly, as just discussed, bringing the correctional officers on board was going to be difficult and she could anticipate resistance from this quarter. In interview with her, Vardon reports a critical moment for her when a prison officer responded to her saying 'why should we help them get educated when you won't educate us?' Her response was to recognize that prison officers too would need education to achieve long term change to their culture and practice.

Consolidation into a larger newly designed prison, with decentralized smaller units of management, was desirable in order to reduce the constant moving of prisoners, to provide continuity of services and staged progression, but this did not occur. Prisons in small communities represent opportunities for permanent work and the threat to close is contentious with electoral ramifications. Other barriers included the primitive state of information technology in the Department at this time which made the adoption of an electronic individual client information system seem heroic in the early stages of the reform process.

Time was needed to appraise resistance to change and figure out effective strategies that could reduce it. Sue Vardon recalls that it was not until 1996 that the responses became clearer. There could not be a single strategy: 'you had to change the environment, you had to get the systems right, you had to get some skills built in and you had to get an understanding of what it was you were doing'. It was a process of learning and a series of shifts in the understanding and practice of people was needed to bring about real organizational cultural change and a new way of doing business.

Vardon realized that this kind of change process had to be led from the top-down. Bottom-up pressure that has been so effective in alliance with top-down reform in driving service reform in areas such as disability services for example (see Handler 1986) was not available in the arena of correctional services. There are limited opportunities for prisoners to be self advocates, their families are rarely advocates on their behalf, and there is next to no support or advocacy from the community or government for such reform. Prisoners may whisper reform, but they don't demand it as there is a fear of payback because 'inside' they have no effective rights, no power, and so much of what goes on inside prison is hidden from external scrutiny.

Vardon in interview also talked about the importance of holding an outsider's perspective but having achieved an insider's credibility in order to provide effective leadership for organizational change. Even while she left the organization at the point at which the pilot process had been completed, her strategic initiation of this reform process was successful and enabled the next stages under a new CEO to engage in its consolidation.

The annual reporting of individualized service reform in SA Correctional Services 1994–2000

The first *Annual Report* under Sue Vardon as CEO covers the period 1993–1994. It indicates that the adoption of the approach of unit management in the prison system has been finalized and guidelines for implementation are in place. Case management is foreshadowed in the strategic priorities (South Australian Department for Correctional Services 1994, 11). At this time the number of prisoners is predicted to increase since 'truth in sentencing' legislation has been enacted and home detention restricted for serious offences. In the 1995–1996 *Annual Report* Vardon's imprint on the Department is fully legible. There is now 'Our Code of Ethics' given pride of place after the 'Mission' statement of the Department. In the Mission statement there is a characteristic Vardon emphasis on the empowering of skilled and committed staff in undertaking the range of services that the Department is charged with providing. In line with Vardon's conviction that an effective organization has to be values-based and values-led, 'Our Code of Ethics' is an explicit values statement that bears the marks of the participatory organizational process that produced it—

> The following Code of Ethics was adopted late in the year and will form the basis of conduct by all staff members in their daily professional lives.
> - *CLIENT FOCUS* We, the staff, will anticipate and be responsive to the individual needs and expectations of clients and other stakeholders with respect and professionalism.
> - *OPTIMISM* We will continue to identify in each individual client their potential to become productive members of society.
> - *TOLERANCE AND IMPARTIALITY* We recognize our task as professionals is to encourage change in each person with whom we have contact and not sit in judgement nor practice or expand any form of punishment which has already been imposed by the courts.
> - *RESPECT* We shall respect every person for their individuality while rejecting and confronting discrimination, prejudice, victimization, physical and psychological bullying and sexual and racial harassment.
> - *CO-OPERATION* We recognize the need for contributions by all staff to the consultative process while accepting and encouraging the creative ability within colleagues to achieve the objective of best practice in all endeavours.
> - *JUSTICE WITH DIGNITY* While supporting the need to provide a safe secure environment for the community, staff will treat all clients in a humane manner while respecting lawful requirements of privacy and confidentiality in discharging their professional duty.

- *HONESTY* Staff feel there is no place in our profession for fraudulent practice, abuse of position or the system.
- *OPENNESS* We will practice open communication with ourselves, clients and the community to guarantee we speak with one voice about our business.
- *ACCOUNTABILITY* All staff will be accountable by: being impartial and competent advisers to clients while efficiently and promptly implementing policies of the Government of the day; being equitable in the discharge of their duty; promoting a safe and healthy work environment; conducting themselves privately in a manner that will not reflect adversely on their employer and avoiding conflicts of interest, real or apparent.

In the same report there is reference to the introduction of a Diploma of Correctional Administration for custodial staff in partnership with the University of South Australia, an initiative designed to professionalize custodial staff training. Throughcare policy, unit management and case management are established as distinct constituents of the new profile of service delivery. 'Throughcare' is defined as the delivery of 'seamless quality service for offenders from initial to final contact'. Case plans are focused on individual need and strategies designed to achieve outcomes for the individual. Case management is the governing instrument for throughcare and case planning. It is represented in the annual report as follows:

> Case management is an individualised service delivery process that is planned and coordinated to achieve throughcare. Adopting a case management approach was one of the most fundamental changes recommended by the review into probation and parole service of the department. In essence case management requires an integrated plan for each defender from reception to termination of contact with the Department. Each offender will be assigned to a case worker who is responsible for the day to day management of an agreed case plan thereby ensuring that throughcare policies are implemented.

By the next *Annual Report* of 1996–1997, there was a new chief executive officer, J.R. Paget. It is clear from this and the next two *Annual Reports* that the direction for reform continued. In the 1996–1997 report, reference is made to ongoing implementation of case management with the Prisoner Assessment Unit identified as the new mechanism

responsible for assessment of individual prisoners and to the introduction of Individual Development Plans. By 1997–1998 the emphasis
is on the consolidation of the case management approach and a service
plan for each prisoner. The CEO reports the first review of the implementation of case management and the new Graduate Certificate
in Case Management to be offered in 1998. The strategies to achieve
throughcare are identified as the quality assurance in case management, system operating procedures to support case management, Individual Development Plans, case reviews, a universal case file which will
become an electronic file to stream line the process (South Australian
Department for Correctional Services 1998, 18–19).

   In the 1998–1999 *Annual Report*, the CEO (still J. R. Paget) to the
Minister indicates that further consolidation of the new case management and throughcare approaches is being undertaken. The reframing
of the prison officer's role as a case officer under the supervision of a
'case coordinator' is also reported:

> In South Australia, similar to most other States, Correctional Officers
> (known as Case Officers) are delivering Case Management services
> to offenders. The Case Officer is supported in the delivery of Case
> Management services by a Case Coordinator and through staff with
> specialist skills providing specialist interventions as required to meet
> the prisoner's needs (South Australian Department for Correctional
> Services 1999, 30).[3]

Additionally, it is reported that the electronic individual client file
began in November 1998 and will become fully operational in 1999/
2000.

   By 2000 Department staff began to present papers about the reforms
in South Australia at national conferences and for the first time outside
of traditional correctional professional forums (Mc Bride 2000). When
Correctional Service presentations were made to the 2000 Case Management Society of Australia conference, for some in the audience the
idea of case management in the corrections arena was viewed as mar-
ginal and even suspect when compared with mainstream applications
of case management in health and welfare. Their suspicion is emblem-
atic of a more general difficulty in bringing the human service professions outside the Corrections arena, as well as the media and general
community, to appreciate the importance of a perspective that locates
Corrections within the wider world of welfare services. Luke Grant,
then Assistant Commissioner for Offender Management, New South

Wales Corrective Services, in interview with Anna Yeatman in 2003 remarked:

> If you rethink what people are doing in custody, and you think ... this is a human service organization [that has] ... regard to the needs and the wellbeing of these people, there should really be no separation in terms of thinking about how we should be able to deliver a service [from] ... any other service delivery organization. ... one of the problems we have is getting any sort of media or other exposure for [the] positive things we do. ... the people who are in my sort of peer group ... have no idea what fabulous people work in the prison system ... All people ... see is the image of a brutal prison officer or ... the graft and bashing of prisoners and they think about assault of prison officers and a punitive ... image of prisons that [was] ... created by Foucault and others that people haven't moved on from.

Evaluating the early stages of case management in South Australian prisons

In 1998 a final year social work group project, under the supervision of Diane Gursansky, was a review of the first six months of the implementation of the case management approach in the South Australian prisons (Burls *et al.* 1998). With the support of senior prison management the students conducted focus groups with prisoners and correctional officers as well as interviews of both prison officers and management at each site. This report was published by the Department. It provides one of the few insights into the distinct perspectives of prisoners, prison officers and prison management on the introduction of the case management approach. Unfortunately it does not include the perspective of specialist staff on the reform process, and this lack is a weakness of this entire case study which should be remedied in further work.

Generally for *prisoners* the new case management approach had come into being, but their individual understanding of case management varied. Most saw the new approach as positive, bringing increased accountability of the prison to them through the case officer and the Individual Development Plan. Prisoners commented on a more civilized and less violent environment since case management had been introduced. They spoke positively about being involved in their assessment and they felt this gave them some individuality. There was a sense of more personal involvement with staff, that staff knew them. Prisoners believed a good case officer is someone who wants to do the job, someone with training to do the job, someone who respects confidentiality and is non-judgemental, approachable, understanding and caring. To make the system work well prisoners stated that they need good information about case management and how it is proposed to work, effective communication with them and their case officers, and a consistent approach to the development and review of case plans. Prisoners also seemed to believe that case plans should be set in place by professional staff. Their concerns were about confidentiality, the actual time available for the case officer to spend with them, and the availability of services to make the plans come alive. Disadvantages of the new approach were linked to concerns about potential personality clashes with case officers, lack of choice in who was the case officer, and especially the dual role of the case officer: 'the screws can't lock you up and be your friend'.

Prison officers who as case officers responded to the review were positive about the new role because it gave new purpose to their work and broke down barriers between officers and prisoners. However on the negative side it was claimed it worked well in theory but broke down in practice. Their concerns matched those of the prisoners: their limited influence as case officers, with prisoners preferring to see the more powerful case manager; the impact of staff shortages on time available to work with individual prisoners; lack of training, and lack of confidence in their own skills to do the job. They also stressed the tension of their dual role and their inadequate training for handling this tension. Completing files was seen as time consuming, meaning more work in an already stretched system. They argued that managers needed to listen to the experience of case officers to shape the new direction. Some asserted that role was too much for them and they were not social workers. They referred to difficulties with maintaining continuity with prisoners who were moved around. Some case officers were seen to avoid their responsibilities by arranging shifts that minimized their involvement with allocated prisoners. Questions were raised about the appropriateness of case management for short term prisoners and people on remand and there was confusion about the role of specialist liaison staff (Aboriginal liaison workers) within the case management system. Most prisoner officers wanted case management to stay but thought further refinement and improvement were necessary. Suggestions for improvement included more formal training, skill development, role definition and clarification.

In the individual interviews with prison officers, they offered thoughtful commentary on case management as a vehicle for cultural change, suggesting that it represented much more than a new practice, and therefore more training and discussion time was needed to help staff rethink their roles. Training in the use of the new file system was seen as imperative. The support of unit managers was essential but it was also noted that specialist staff needed to more effectively include case officers in processes and decision making. There was a sense that all the attention was focused on changing custodial staff practice without recognizing that other specialist staff also needed to adapt their practices if they were to work in collaboration with case officers and case managers. Custodial officers talked about there needing to be incentives for prisoners to engage in case management.

Staff rostering so as to permit pairing of staff with prisoners was seen to be a critical factor. The most critical issue was consistently that of the conflicting roles of custodial and helping. Overlaying this issue was the industrial concerns with extra demands beyond their negotiated responsibilities. Some individual staff who declared a very positive response to the new opportunities offered through case management, expressed the view that they needed to be cautious in the presence of many colleagues who were quite resistant to the changes. Building a team approach to case management both in the unit and across the department was seen as critical to the process and the response of professional staff to sharing knowledge with custodial staff was identified as a major block. They did not argue they needed access to all personal details but they did need to be kept informed of changing circumstances to be effective in their interactions with the prisoner. For some case management represented another example of a new idea that would never be fully implemented. Those opposed to the changes declared openly they did not want to move away from the custodial role. However those who supported the shift wanted to build skills and become more knowledgeable about resources to assist prisoners.

From a *management* perspective it was hardly surprising to find the endorsement of the shift. The declared advantages of the of case management were improved relationships with prisoners, reduced number of incidents, increased accountability, and more personalized service delivery. At the same time, continuing issues included the skill base of prison officers, the intensification of work demands on them, and the high expectations of the case management approach. As with the prison officers, the managers supported the need for training, clarification of confidentiality walls in files, and for the sustaining of individual case plans. Managers recognized that, as long the service system is arranged around the needs of staff, the needs of prisoners would be neglected, and this is what case management is challenging.

Conclusion

This chapter reports the early phases of significant reform in the individualizing of correctional services, and thereby bringing them within the mainstream ethos of contemporary human services, in one case: that of the South Australian Department of Correctional Services in the period of 1993 to 2000. The case study is significant not only for the possibilities and difficulties it indicates in bringing the area of correctional services into an individualized human service approach, but for the window it offers on the way in which the individual leadership of a visionary and reform-oriented public servant can make a significant difference to the pace and trajectory of reform.

Notes

1   The change in 1974 of the title of the government department responsible for this area in South Australia is suggestive of this era of change: from being known as The Prison's Department, it was renamed as The Department of Correctional Services. It is now known as the Department for Correctional Services.

2   They continue: 'In short, offending can reflect the search for certain kinds of experience, namely, the attainment of specific goals or goods. Furthermore, offenders' personal strivings express their sense of who they are and what they would like to become. Narrative identities, for offenders and for all people, are constituted from the pursuit and achievement of personal goals. This feature of offending renders it more intelligible and, in a sense, more human. It reminds us that effective treatment should aim to provide alternative methods for achieving human goods' (Ward and Marshall 2007, 279). For a case study of this approach to someone who is a high-risk violent offender, see Whitehead, Ward and Collie (2007).

3   This is in line with an interview undertaken later in 2003 (by Anna Yeatman) with the Assistant Commissioner, Offender Management in the New South Wales Department of Corrective Services, who said that as of this time prison officers are not educated enough to be the case managers. Instead they are called 'case officers' who will work with a new classification of worker; instead of specialist classifications such as welfare officers, drug and alcohol officers, there was to be a services and programs officer who undertook the role of case planning and case management.

Consolidated Bibliography

Abbey, J., K. Frogatt, D. Parker and B. Abbey 'Palliative care in long-term care: a system in change', *International Journal of Older People Nursing*, 1, 56–63.

Althaus, C. (1997) 'The application of agency theory to public sector management', in G. Davis, B. Sullivan and A. Yeatman (eds) *The New Contractualism?* South Melbourne: Macmillan Education Australia, 137–154.

Alvarez, A. (2002) *Live Company*: *Psychoanalytic Psychotherapy with Autistic, Borderline, Deprived and Abused Children*, East Sussex and New York: Brunner-Routledge.

Arendt, H. (1975) *The Origins of Totalitarianism*, San Deigo, New York and London: Harcourt Brace Jovanovich (Harvest Book).

Arendt, H. (1994) 'Understanding and Politics (The Difficulties of Understanding)', in *Essays in Understanding 1930–1954* (ed. Jerome Kohn), New York, San Diego and London: Harcourt Brace, 307–328.

Arendt, H. (2005) 'Socrates' in *The Promise of Politics* (ed. Jerome Kohn), New York: Schocken Books.

Ariss, R., G. Dowsett and T. Carrigan (1995) 'Health Strategies of HIV-Infected, Homosexually Active Men in Sydney', *Journal of Gay & Lesbian Social Services*, 3 (3), 49–71.

Austin, C. and R. McClelland (eds) (1996) *Perspectives on Case Management Practice*, Milwaukee: Families International.

Australian Institute of Health and Welfare (2001) 'Deinstitutionalisation', *Australia's Welfare, 2001*, Canberra: AIHW, 96–139.

Australian Institute of Health and Welfare (2003a) *Community Aged Care Packages in Australia 2001–02: a statistical overview, Aged Care Statistics Series no. 14*, Cat No. 30, Australian Institute of Health and Welfare, Canberra.

Australian Institute of Health and Welfare (2003b) *Australia's Welfare 2003*, Canberra: AIHW.

Australian Institute of Health and Welfare (2004) *Community Aged Care Packages Census 2002*, Cat. No. AGE 35, Canberra: AIHW.

Australian Institute of Health and Welfare (2005) *Australia's Welfare 2005*, Canberra: AIHW.

Australian Institute of Health and Welfare (2007) *Aged Care Packages in the Community 2005–06: a statistical overview, Aged Care Statistics Series No. 25*, Cat. No. 55, Canberra: AIHW.

Australian Senate (1985) *Private Nursing Homes in Australia: their conduct, administration and ownership*, Senate Select Committee on Private Hospitals and Nursing Homes, Canberra: AGPS.

Ballard, J. (1998) 'The Constitution of AIDS in Australia: Taking 'Government at a Distance' Seriously', in M. Dean and B. Hindess (eds) *Governing Australia: Studies in Contemporary Rationalities of Government*, Cambridge: Cambridge University Press, 125–139.

Barnardos Australia (2006) *Annual Review 2005/06*, Sydney: Barnardos Australia.

Barnes, M. (1999) 'Users as Citizens: Collective Action and the Local Governance of Welfare', *Social Policy & Administration*, 33 (1), 73–90.

Batrouney, C. (1999) 'Once were warriors: how activism was cured before AIDS', *HIV Herald*, 8 (6), 3–19.

Batrouney, C. and L. Crooks (1998) 'You are not alone: access a positive diagnosis' (information booklet) Sydney: AFAO/ACON—no pagination.

Beck, A. (1999) 'Trends in US Correctional Populations', in K. Haas and G. Alpert *The Dilemma of Corrections: Contemporary Readings*, Prospect Heights, Illinois: Waveland Press, 44–65.

Bell, M. (1998/1999) 'The Looking After Children Materials: A critical analysis of their use in practice', *Adoption and Fostering*, 22 (4), 15–23.

Benjamin, J. (2004) 'Beyond Doer and Done To: an Intersubjective View of Thirdness', *Psychoanalytic Quarterly*, LXXIII, 5–47.

Bennington, L. and J. Cummane (1997) 'Customer Driven Research: The Customer Value Workshop', in P. Kunst and J. Lemmink (eds) *Managing Service Quality*, 111, 89–106.

Beresford, P. (2001) 'Service users, social policy and the future of welfare', *Critical Social Policy*, 21 (4), 494–512.

Bigby, C. and C. Fyffe (2006) 'Tensions between institutional closure and deinstitutionalisation: what can be learned from Victoria's institutional redevelopment?', *Disability & Society*, 21 (6), 567–561.

Bigby, C. and E. Ozanne (2001) 'Shifts in the model of service delivery in intellectual disability in Victoria', *Journal of Intellectual & Developmental Disability*, 26 (2), 177–190.

Bion, W. (1994) *Learning from Experience*, New Jersey and London: Jason Aronson.

Bird, G. (2002) 'Prisoners of Difference', in D. Brown and M. Wilkie (eds) *Prisoners as Citizens: Human Rights in Australian Prisons*, Leichhardt, New South Wales: The Federation Press, 65–78.

Bollas, C. (1989) *Forces of Destiny: Psychoanalysis and Human Idiom*, London: Free Association Books.

Bollas, C. (1993) *Being a Character: Psychoanalysis and Self Experience*, London: Routledge.

Bollas, C. (1999) 'The place of the psychoanalyst', in *The Mystery of Things*, London: Routledge, 15–27.

Bollas, C. (2001) 'Dead mother, dead child', in G. Kohon (ed.) *The Dead Mother: The Work of André Green*, Hove and Philadelphia: Brunner-Routledge, 87–109.

Bollas, C. (2007) *The Freudian Moment*, London: Karnac.

Boston, J., J. Martin, J. Pallot and P. Walsh (1996) *Public Management: the New Zealand Model*, Oxford: Oxford University Press.

Braithwaite, J. (1998) 'Institutionalizing distrust, enculturating trust', in V. Braithwaite and M. Levi (eds) *Trust and Governance*, New York: Russell Sage, 343–381.

Braithwaite, J. and T. Makkai (1994) 'Trust and compliance', *Policing and Society*, 4, 1–12.

Braithwaite, J., T. Makkai and V. Braithwaite (2007) *Regulating Aged Care: Ritualism and the New Pyramid*, Cheltenham, UK and Northampton, MA, USA: Edward Elgar.

Briggs, A. (2002) *Surviving Space: Papers on Infant Observation*, London and New York, Karnac.

Brown, D. and M. Wilkie (eds) (2002) *Prisoners as Citizens: Human Rights in Australia*, Leichhardt, New South Wales: The Federation Press.

Burchard, J.D. and R.T. Clarke (1990) 'The Role of Individualized Care in a Service Delivery System for Children and Adolescents with Severely Maladjusted Behaviour', *The Journal of Mental Health Administration*, 17 (1): 48–60.

Burls, K., D. Cleaver, C. Griffiths, C. Jukes, C. Kulas, B. Lynch, B. Mahar, J. Oake, S. Phillips, J. Purtle and N. Zweck (1998) *Review of Case Management … stakeholders' views*, a project undertaken by BSW students from the School of Social Work and Social Policy, University of South Australia for the South Australian Department of Correctional Services, Adelaide.

CACP Guidelines (1999) *Community Care Packages Program Guidelines*, Canberra: Department of Health and Ageing.

CACP Guidelines (2004) *Community Care Packages Program Guidelines*, Canberra: Department of Health and Ageing http://www.health.gov.au/internet/wcms/publishing.nsf/Content/ageing-commcare-comcprov-ccpindex.htm/$FILE/ccpguide.pdf downloaded Nov 2004.

Campbell, J., L. Brophy, B. Healy and A. O'Brien (2006) 'International Perspectives on the Use of Community Treatment Orders: Implications for Mental Health Social Workers', *British Journal of Social Work* 36, 1101–1118.

Capitman, J.A., B. Haskins and J. Bernstein (1986) 'Case management approaches in coordinated community-oriented long-term demonstrations', *The Gerontologist,* 26 (4), 398–404.

Carlson, P. (1999) 'The Legacy of Punishment', in P. Carlson and J. Garrett (eds) *Prison and Jail Administration: Practice and Theory*, Maryland, USA: Aspen Publishers, 3–6.

Carlson, P. and J. Garrett (1999) *Prison and Jail Administration: Practice and Theory*, Maryland, USA: Aspen Publishers.

Carnaby, S. (1997) 'A Comparative Approach to Evaluating Individual Planning for People with Learning Disabilities', *Disability and* Society, 12(3) 381–394.

Carr, S. (2007) 'Participation, power, conflict and change: Theorizing dynamics of service user participation in the social care system of England and Wales', *Critical Social Policy*, 27 (2), 266–276.

Cashmore, J. and F. Ainsworth (2004) *Audit of Australian Out-of-Home Care Research*, Sydney: Association of Childrens Welfare Agencies Inc. http://www.acwa.asn.au/cafwaa/ResearchAudit2004.pdf

Cashmore, J., R. Dolby and D. Brennan (1994) *Systems Abuse: Problems and Solutions*, Sydney: NSW Child Protection Council.

Centrelink (1999) *Centrelink Annual Report 1998–1999*, Commonwealth of Australia.

Centrelink (2001) *Centrelink Annual Review 2000–2001*, ACT, Australia: Centrelink.

Centrelink (2003) *Centrelink Annual Review 2002–2003*, ACT, Australia: Canberra Business Centre.

Centrelink (2004) 'Resignation of Sue Vardon', National Media Release—http://www.centrelink.gov.au/internet/internet.nsf/news_room/04natio...

Centrelink (2005) *Centrelink Annual Report 2004–2005*, Centrelink, ACT, Australia: Canberra Business Centre.

Clare, M. (1997) 'The UK "Looking After Children" Project Fit for "out-of-home care" Practice in Australia?', *Children Australia*, 22, 29–35.

Clark, C. (1998) Self-determination and Paternalism in Community Care: Practice and Prospects, *Br J Social Work*, 28 (3), 387–402.

Clarke, R. and G. Burke (1998) *'Looking After Children': An Evaluation of the Victorian Pilot Program*, Children's Welfare Association of Victoria Research Paper.

Cohen, B. (2002) 'Alternative Organizing Principles for the Design of Service Delivery Systems', *Administration in Social Work*, 26 (2), 17–39.

Comas-Herrera, A., R. Wittenberg and L. Pickard (2004) 'Long-term care for older people in the United Kingdom: structure and challenges', in M. Knapp, D. Challis, J.-L. Fernández and A. Netten (2004*) Long-Term Care: Matching Resources and Needs*, Aldershot: Ashgate, 17–35.

Commonwealth of Australia (2005) *National HIV/AIDS Strategy: Revitalising Australia's Response 2005–2008*, Canberra.

Cooper, A. and J. Lousada (2005) *Borderline Welfare: Feeling and Fear of Feeling in Modern Welfare*, London and New York: Karnac.

Cowden, S. and G. Singh (2007) 'The "User": Friend, foe or fetish? A critical exploration of user involvement in health and social care', *Critical Social Policy* 27 (1), 5–23.

Crooks, L. (1989) 'The needs of HIV infected persons: impressions from the Wollongong AIDS research project in light of recent calls for people to "come out"', *National Aids Bulletin*, December, 18–23.

Crow, I. (2001) *The Treatment and Rehabilitation of Offenders*, London: Sage.

Danley, K. and V. Mellen (1987) 'Training and Personal Issues for Supported Employment Programs which Serve Persons who are Severely Mentally Ill', *Psychosocial Rehabilitation Journal*, 11 (2), 87–102.

Dant, T. and B. Gearing (1990) 'Keyworkers for elderly people in the community: case managers and care co-ordinators', *Journal of Social Policy*, 19 (3), 331–360.

Davies, B.P. (1994) 'Improving the case management process', in *Caring for Frail Elderly People: 1. New Direction in Care*, Paris: OECD, 111–143.

Davies, R. (1994) *A Cunning Man*, Penguin Books.

Davis, A. (2001) 'Labelled encounters and experiences: ways of seeing, thinking about and responding to uniqueness', *Nursing Philosophy*, 2, 101–111.

Davis, M. and D. Wallbridge (1981) *Boundary and Space: an Introduction to the Work of D.W. Winnicott*, London: Karnac Books.

Dawes, J. (2002) 'Institutional Perspectives and Constraints', in Brown, D. and M. Wilkie (eds) *Prisoners as Citizens: Human Rights in Australian Prisons*, Leichhardt, New South Wales: The Federation Press, 115–130.

Daye, J. (2001) 'Emotional Health and Well Being: Breaking Down the Barriers', Proceedings of the 8th National Conference of People Living with HIV/AIDS, 1–5.

DCS (1986) *Nursing Homes and Hostels Review*, Department of Community Services, AGPS, Canberra.

De Jong, P. and I. Berg (2001) 'Co-Constructing Cooperation with Mandated Clients', *Social Work*, 46 (4), 361–375.

De Schweinitz, K. (1943/1961) *England's Road to Social Security*, New York: A S Barnes-Perpetua Edition.

DEWR (2005) *Annual Report 2004–2005*, Department of Employment and Workplace Relations, Commonwealth of Australia.

DHHCS (1991) *Aged Care Reform Strategy Mid Term Review 1990–1991*, Department of Health Housing and Community Services, Canberra: Australian Government Publishing Service.

DHSH (1995) *The Efficiency and Effectiveness Review of the Home and Community Care Program. Final Report*, Aged And Community Care Division, Service Development and Evaluation Reports No. 18, Canberra: Australian Government Publishing Service.

Dickerson, F. (1998) 'Strategies that Foster Empowerment', *Cognitive and Behavioural Practice*, 5, 255–275.

Dickey, B. (1980) *No Charity There. A Short History of Social Welfare in Australia*, Melbourne: Thomas Nelson.

Dixon, D. (2001) 'Looking After Children in Barnardos Australia: a study of the early stages of implementation', *Children Australia* 26 (3), 27–33.

Dixon, D. and J. Morwitzer (2001) *Pitfalls, not just Positives*, Presentation by The LAC Project to the Face to Face LAC and Quality Forum, UNSW, 20th August 2001, unpublished paper.

Dowden, C. and D. Andrews (2000) 'Effective Correctional Treatment and Violent Re-offending: a meta-analysis', *Canadian Journal of Criminology*, 42, 444–467.

Dowsett, G. (1996) 'Perspectives in Australian HIV/AIDS Health Promotion', in NSW HIV/AIDS Health Promotion Conference: Keynote Addresses, Selected Papers and Future Directions, comp. NSW AIDS/Infectious Diseases Branch, NSW Health Publication (AIDS) 96-0067, Sydney, 19–31.

Dowsett, G. (1998) 'Pink Conspiracies: Australia's Gay Communities and National HIV/AIDS Policies', in A. Yeatman (ed.) *Activism and the Policy Process*, St Leonards: Allen & Unwin, 171–194.

Dowsett, G. (2003) 'HIV/AIDS and homophobia: subtle hatreds, severe consequences and the question of origins', *Culture, Health & Sexuality*, 5 (2), 121–136.

Dowsett, G. (2006) 'Brokeback to Bareback: Shifts in Gay Sexual Culture and Dilemmas for Prevention Research', Opening Plenary Address, *Stigma/Pleasure/Practice: the 9th Social Research Conference on HIV*, Hepatitis C and Related Diseases, University of New South Wales, Sydney, 20–21 April.

Dowsett, G. and D. McInnes (1996) 'Gay community, AIDS agencies and the HIV epidemic in Adelaide: theorising the "post-AIDS"', *Social Alternatives*, 15 (4), 29–32.

Dowsett, G., J. Bollen, D. McInnes, M. Couch and B. Edwards (2001) 'HIV/AIDS and constructs of gay community: researching educational practice within community-based health promotion for gay men', *Social Research Methodology* 4 (3), 2005–2223.

Du Gay, P. (2000) *In Praise of Bureaucracy: Weber-Organization-Ethics*, London, Thousand Oaks and New Delhi: Sage.

Du Gay, P. (2005) 'Bureaucracy and Liberty: State, Authority and Freedom', in P. Du Gay (ed.) *The Values of Bureaucracy*, Oxford: Oxford University Press, 41–63.

Durkheim, É. (1964) *The Division of Labor in Society*, New York: Free Press.

Feenan, R. (2000) 'Implementing Case Management in NSW Corrections: An Exercise in Change Management', Presentation at the Case Management Society of Australia Conference, February, Melbourne, Australia.

Feinberg, L. and C. Ellano (2000) 'Promoting Consumer Direction for Family Caregiver Support: an Agency-Driven Model', *Generations*, Fall, 47–54.

Feldenkrais, M. (1990) *Awareness through Movement: Health Exercises for Personal Growth*, Arkana Penguin Books.

Ferguson, H. (2001) 'Social Work, Individualization and Life Politics', *British Journal of Social Work*, 31, 41–55.

Ferguson, H. (2003) 'In Defence (and Celebration) of Individualization and Life Politics for Social Work', *British Journal of Social Work*, 33, 699–707.

Ferguson, H. (2007) 'Abused and Looked After Children as "Moral Dirt": Child Abuse and Institutional Care in Historical Perspective', *Journal of Social Policy*, 36: 1, 123–139.

Ferguson, I. (2007) 'Increasing User Choice or Privatizing Risk? The Antinomies of Personalization', *British Journal of Social Work*, 37, 387–403.

Fernández, J.-L., J. Kendall, V. Davey and M. Knapp (2007) Direct Payments in England: Factors Linked to Variations in Local Provision, *Journal of Social Policy* 36 (1), 97–121.

Fine, M. (1998) 'Acute and Continuing Care for Older People in Australia: Contesting New Balances of Care', in C. Glendinning (ed.) *Rights and Realities: Comparing New Developments in Long-Term Care for Older People*, Bristol: The Policy Press, 105–126.

Fine, M. (1999) 'Ageing and the balance of responsibilities between the various providers of child and aged care: shaping policies for the future', in *Policy Implications of the Ageing of Australia's Population*, Conference Proceedings, Canberra: Ausinfo.

Fine, M. (2005a) 'Dependency Work. A critical exploration of Kittay's perspective on care as a relationship of power', *Health Sociology Review*, 14 (2), 146–160.

Fine, M. (2005b) 'Individualisation, risk and the body. Sociology and care', *Journal of Sociology*, 41 (3), 249–268.

Fine, M. and J. Chalmers (2000) 'User Pays and Other Approaches to the Funding of Long-Term Care for Older People in Australia', *Ageing and Society* 20 (1), 5–32.

Fine, M. and C. Glendinning (2005) 'Dependence, independence or interdependence? Revisiting the concepts of "care" and "dependency"', *Ageing and Society*, 25 (4), 601–621.

Fine, M. and J. Stevens (1998) 'From inmates to consumers: developments in Australian aged care since white settlement', in B. Jeawoddy and C. Saw (ed.) *Successful Aging. Perspectives on Health and Social Construction*, Sydney, Mosby: 39–92.

Fisher, K. and M. Fine (2002) 'Care Coordination, Case Management Theory and the Coordinated Care Trials. Reconsidering the Fundamentals', *The Australian Coordinated Care Trials: Reflection on the Evaluation (Vol. 2)*, Canberra: Department of Health and Ageing, 23–39.

Fiumara, C. (1990) *The Other Side of Language: a Philosophy of Listening*, London and New York: Routledge.

Flaskas, C. (2007) 'The Balance of Hope and Hopelessness', in C. Flaskas, I. McCarthy and J. Sheehan (eds) *Hope and Despair in Narrative and Family Therapy: Adversity, Forgiveness and Reconciliation*, London and New York: Routledge, 24–36.

Fonagy, P., G. Gergely, E. Jurist and M. Target (2004) *Affect Regulation, Mentalization and the Development of the Self*, London and New York: Karnac.

Fox, D.M. and C. Raphael (eds) (1997) *Home-Based Care for a New Century*, Blackwell, Malden MA.

Gibson, D.M. (1998) *Aged Care: Old Policies, New Solutions*, Melbourne: Cambridge University Press.

Gibson, D. and S. Mathur (1999) 'Australian innovations in home-based care: a comparison of Community Aged Care Packages, Community Options and Hostel Care', *Australasian Journal of Ageing*, 18 (2): 72–78.

Glendinning, C., S. Halliwell, S. Jacobs, K. Rummery and J. Tyrer (2000) 'New kinds of care, new kinds of relationships: how purchasing services affects relationships in giving and receiving personal assistance', *Health & Social Care in the Community*, 8 (3), 201–211.

Goffman, E. (1968) *Asylums*, Harmondsworth, Pelican.

Gordon, R. (1985) 'Macaulay, Macneil and the Discovery of Solidarity and Power in Contract Law', *Wisconsin Law Review*, 563–580.

Grierson, J., S. Misson, K. McDonald, M. Pitts and M. O'Brien (2002) *HIV Futures 3: Positive Australians on Services, Health and Well-Being*, The Living with HIV Program, La Trobe University: Australian Research Centre in Sex, Health and Society, Monograph Series Number 37, May.

Gursansky, D., J. Harvey, and R. Kennedy (2003) *Case Management: Policy, Practice and Professional Business*, Crows Nest, New South Wales: Allen & Unwin.

Halligan, J. (2006) 'Interagency Management of Service Delivery in a Complex Environment: the case of Centrelink', in Colin Campbell et al. *Comparative Trends in Public Management: Smart Practices Towards Blending Policy and Administration*, Ottawa, Canada: Canada School of Public Service, 86–106.

Handler, J. (1986) *The Conditions of Discretion: Autonomy, Community, Bureaucracy*, New York: Russell Sage Foundation.

Harris, J. (1999) 'State Social Work and Social Citizenship in Britain: from clientelism to Consumerism', *British Journal of Social Work*, 29, 915–937.

Hasenfeld, Y. (1992) 'The Nature of Human Service Organisations', in Y. Hasenfeld (ed.) *Human Services as Complex Organizations*, Newbury Park, London and New Delhi: Sage, 3–24.

Hass, K.C. and Alpert, G.P. (1999) *The Dilemmas of Corrections: Contemporary Readings*, Prospect Heights, Illinois, USA: Waveland Press.

Hegel, G. (1991) *Elements of the Philosophy of Right*, Cambridge: Cambridge University Press.

Herman, J. (2001) *Trauma and Recovery: From Domestic Abuse to Political Terror*, London: Pandora.

Heyes, C. (2007) *Self-Transformations: Foucault, Ethics, and Normalized Bodies*, Oxford: Oxford University Press.

Hirst, D. and P. Michael (2003) 'Family, Community and the "Idiot" in Mid-nineteenth Century North Wales', *Disability & Society*, 18 (2), 145–163.

Hogg, R. (2002) 'Prisoners and the Penal Estate in Australia', in D. Brown and M. Wilkie (eds) *Prisoners as Citizens: Human Rights in Australian Prisons*, Leichhardt, New South Wales: Federation Press, 3–20.

Hoggett, P. (2000) *Emotional Life and the Politics of Welfare*, Basingstoke and London: Macmillan.

Hoggett, P. (2001) 'Agency, Rationality and Social Policy', *Journal of Social Policy*, 30(1), 37–56.

Hoggett, P. (2005a) 'Democracy, Government and Emotional Experience', paper presented to 'Governed States of Mind', a joint Tavistock/Open University conference, St Hilda's College, Oxford University (to be partially incorporated in Hoggett's forthcoming book *Politics, Identity and Emotion*, Paradigm Publishers, 2008).

Hoggett, P. (2005b) 'A Service to the Public: the Containment of Ethical and Moral Conflicts by Public Bureaucracies', in P. Du Gay (ed.) *The Values of Bureaucracy*, Oxford: Oxford University Press, 165–191.

Hoggett, P. (2008) 'Relational Thinking and Welfare Practice', in S. Clarke, H. Hahn and P. Hoggett (eds) *Object Relations and Social Relations*, London: Karnac.

Home and Community Care Review Working Group (1988) *First Triennial Review of the Home and Community Care Program*, Canberra: Australian Government Publishing Service.

Hopkins, K. and C. Hyde (2002) 'The Human Service Managerial Dilemma: New Expectations, Chronic Challenges and Old Solutions', *Administration in Social Work*, 26 (3), 1–16.

Houston, J. (1999) *Correctional Management: Functions, Skills and Systems*, Chicago: Nelson-Hall Publishers.

Howard, C. (2006) 'The new governance of Australian welfare: street-level contingencies', in P. Henman and M. Fenger (eds) *Administering Welfare Reform: International transformations in welfare governance*, University of Bristol: the Policy Press, 137–161.

Howe, A. (1997) 'The Aged Care Reform Strategy: a decade of changing momentum and margins for reform', in A. Borowski, S. Encel and E. Ozanne (eds) *Ageing and Social Policy in Australia*, Melbourne: Cambridge University Press, 301–326.

Hunter, I. (2001) *Rival Enlightenments: Civil and Metaphysical Philosophy in Early Modern Germany*, Cambridge: Cambridge University Press.

Independent Commission Against Corruption (ICAC) (1999) *Case Management in New South Wales Correctional Centres*, Sydney: ICAC.

Isaacs, S. (1989) 'The Nature and Function of Phantasy', in M. Klein, P. Heimann, S. Isaacs and J. Riviere *Developments in Psychoanalysis*, London: Karnac Books, 67–122.

Jackson, S. (1998) 'Looking After Children: a new approach or just an exercise in formfilling? A response to Knight and Caveney', *British Journal of Social Work* 28, 45–56.

Jalland, P. (2005) 'Changing Ways of Grieving in 20th Century Australia', *Dialogue*, Academy of the Social Sciences of Australia, 24 (3), 4–19.

Jones, K. and A. Fowles (1984) *Ideas on Institutions. Analysing the literature on long-term care and custody*, London: Routledge & Kegan Paul.

Jones, H., R. Clark, K. Kufeldt and M. Norrman (1998) 'Looking After Children: Assessing outcomes in Child Care. The Experience of implementation', *Children & Society*, 12 (3), 201–222.

Jopson, D. and A. Horin (2007) 'Pursuit of the poor under review', The Sydney Morning Herald, December 11 http://www.smh.com.au/cgi-bin/common/popupPrintArticle.pl?path=/a...

Kapp, M. (1997) 'Control versus Consent in Community-Based Long-term Care Services: the role of economic empowerment', *International Journal of Economic Empowerment* 20 (2), 295–307.

Kearns, R. with Bernice and Margaret (1996) 'Using the LOOKING AFTER CHILDREN Assessment and Action Records', *Child Care in Practice*, 2 (4), 83–86.

Keating, M. (2001) 'Reshaping Service Delivery', in G. Davis and P. Weller (eds) *Are You Being Served? State, Citizens and Governance*, Crows Nest: Allen & Unwin, 98–126.

Keigher, S. (1999) 'The Limits of Consumer Directed Care as Public Policy in an Aging Society', *Canadian Journal on Aging*, 18 (2), 182–210.

266 *Consolidated Bibliography*

Kendrick, M. (2002) 'When people matter more than systems', Keynote Present-
ation for Conference *The Promise of Opportunity*, Albany, New York, March
27–28, 2000.
Kingdom, E. (2000) 'Cohabitation Contracts and the Democratization of Per-
sonal Relations', *Feminist Legal Studies*, 8: 5–27.
Kippax, S. and K. Race (2003) 'Sustaining Safe Practice: Twenty Years On', *Social
Science & Medicine*, 57 (1), 1–12.
Kittay, E. (1999) *Love's Labor: Essays on Women, Equality, and Dependency*, New
York: Routledge.
Kittay, E. (2001) 'A Feminist Public Ethic of Care Meets the New Commun-
itarian Family Policy', *Ethics*, 111 (April), 523–547.
Kotter, J. (1995) 'Leading Change: Why Transformation Efforts Fail', *Harvard
Business Review*, March–April, 59–68.
Kriegel, B. (1995) *The State and the Rule of Law*, translated by M. LePain and
J. Cohen, Princeton NJ: Princeton University Press.
Lauen, R. (1994) *Positive Approaches to Corrections Research, Policy and Practice,*
Lanham, Maryland: American Correctional Association.
Levine, D. (1995) *Wealth and Freedom: an introduction to political economy*, Cam-
bridge: Cambridge University Press.
Liebling, A. (2003) 'Moral Values, Prison Performance and the Problem of Quality:
a Summary and Discussion Paper', Cambridge Institute of Criminology, unpub-
lished paper.
Locke, J. (1970) *Two Treatises of Government*, Cambridge: Cambridge University
Press.
McBride, J. (2000) 'Case Management in South Australian Prisons', Presentation
at the Case Management Society of Australia Conference, February, Melbourne,
Australia.
McCallum, S. (2002) 'Social Work in the Era of Case Management', in P. Swain
(ed.) *In the Shadow of the Law: The Legal Context of Social Work Practice*, Second
Edition, Leichhardt, New South Wales, The Federation Press, 61–71.
McCallum, S. and J. Furby (1999) 'Case Management for the NT Correctional
Services', *Australian Social Work*, 52 (4), 45–49.
McCormack, B. (2002) 'The Person of the Voice: Narrative Identities in Informed
Consent', *Nursing Philosophy* 3, 114–119.
McCormack, B. (2004) 'Person-centredness in gerontological nursing: an
overview of the literature', *International Journal of Older People Nursing*, 13,
31–38.
McLeay, L. (1982) *In a Home or At Home: Accommodation and Home Care for the
Aged,* Report of the House of Representatives Standing Committee on Expend-
iture (Chaired by L. McLeay), Canberra: AGPS.
Machon, K. (2002) Paper for the HIV Retrospectives Conference (no title), Uni-
versity of New South Wales, May.
Maddocks, I. (2005) 'Death and Dying in Australia—the Contribution of
Palliative Care', *Dialogue*, Academy of the Social Sciences of Australia, 24 (3),
46–58.
Malpas, J. (2007) 'Human Dignity and Human Being', in J. Malpas and N. Lickiss
(eds) *Perspectives on Human Dignity: A Conversation*, Dordrecht: Springer, 19–26.
Maluccio, A and W. Marlow (1974) 'The Case of Contract', *Social Work*, 19: 1,
28–38.

Mathur, S., A. Evans and D. Gibson (1997) *Community Aged Care Packages. How do they compare?*, Aged and Community Care Service Development and Evaluation Reports No. 32, Canberra: Commonwealth Department of Health and Family Services.

Mead, L. (1997) 'The Rise of Paternalism', in L. Mead (ed.) *The New Paternalism: Supervisory Approaches to Poverty*, Brookings Institute Press, Washington DC.

Mead, L. (2005) 'Welfare Reform and Citizenship', in L. Mead and C. Beem (eds) *Welfare Reform and Political Theory*, New York: Russell Sage Foundation.

Mead, L. and C. Beem (eds) (2005) *Welfare Reform and Political Theory*, New York: Russell Sage Foundation.

Menadue, D. 'Lipo: Any Progress?', from *Positive Living*, 1 December, on the NAPWA website—www.napwa.org.au/node/655

Mendes, P. and B. Moslehuddin (2004) 'Graduating from the child welfare system: a comparison of the UK and Australian leaving care debates', *International Journal of Social Welfare*, 13, 332–329.

Mitrani, J. (2001) *Ordinary People and Extra-Ordinary Protections: A Post-Kleinian Approach to the Treatment of Primitive Mental States*, Hove and New York: Brunner-Routledge.

Monahan, J., R. Bonnie, P. Appelbaum, P. Hyde, H. Steadman and M. Swartz (2001) 'Mandated Community Treatment: Beyond Outpatient Commitment', *Psychiatric Services*, 52 (9), 1198–1206.

Moore, A. (2005) 'Modelling Agency in HIV Treatment Decision Making', *Australian Review of Applied Linguistics*, Special Edition, S19, 103–122.

Morris, J. (1997) 'Care or Empowerment? A Disability Rights Perspective', *Social Policy & Administration*, 31 (1), 54–60.

Moxley, D. (1997) *Case Management by Design: Reflections on principles and practices*, Chicago: Nelson Hall.

Nedelsky, J. (1990) 'Law, Boundaries and the Bounded Self', *Representations*, 30, 162–190.

Nedelsky, J. (1993) 'Reconceiving Rights as Relationship', *Review of Constitutional Studies*, 1 (1), 1–27.

New South Wales Department of Community Services (2006) *Annual Report 2005/6*, [online] Available at: http://www.community.nsw.gov.au/documents/annual_report05–06.

Niven, C. and P. Scott (2003) 'The need for accurate perception and informed judgement in determining the appropriate use of the nursing resource: hearing the patient's voice', *Nursing Philosophy*, 4, 201–210.

Nolan, L. (2006) 'Caring connections with older persons with dementia in an acute hospital setting—a hermeneutic interpretation of the staff nurse's experience', *International Journal of Older People Nursing*, 1, 208–215.

Noring, S., N. Dubler, G. Birkhead and B. Agins (2001) 'A New Paradigm for HIV Care: Ethical and Clinical Considerations', *American Journal of Public Health*, 91 (5), 690–695.

Novak, J., D. Mank, G. Revell and D. O'Brien (1999) 'Paying for Success: Results-Based Approaches to Funding Supported Employment', in Revell, Inge, Mank and Wehmen (eds) *The Impact of Supported Employment on People with Significant Disabilities: Preliminary Findings of the National Supported Employment Consortium* Richmond, VA: Virginia Commonwealth University Rehabilitation Research and Training Center on Workplace Supports.

Nussbaum, M. (1986) 'Non-scientific Deliberation', in *The Fragility of Goodness: Luck and Ethics in Greek Tragedy and Philosophy*, Cambridge: Cambridge University Press, 290–318.

Ogden, T. (1996) *Subjects of Analysis*, Northvale, N.J. and London: Jason Aronson.

Ogden, T. (2008) 'On holding and containing, being and dreaming', in L. Caldwell (ed.) *Winnicott and the Psychoanalytic Tradition*, London: Karnac, 76–97.

Ozanne, E. (1990) 'Reasons for the Emergence of Case Management Approaches and their Distinctiveness from Present Service Arrangements', in A. Howe, E. Ozanne and C. Selby Smith (eds) *Community Care Policy and Practice: New Directions in Australia*, Monash University, Clayton Victoria: Public Sector Institute, 186–195.

Palmer, T. (1999) 'The Effectiveness Issue Today', in K. Hass and G. Alpert (eds) *The Dilemma of Corrections: Contemporary Readings*, Prospect Heights, Illinois: Waveland Press, 339–354.

Parker, R. (1998) 'Reflection on the Assessment of Outcomes in Child Care', *Children & Society*, 12 (1998), 192–201.

Parsons, T. (1951) *The Social System*, London, Routledge and Kegan Paul.

Parsons, T. (1957) 'Illness and the Role of the Physician: A Sociological Perspective', *American Journal of Orthopsychiatry*, 21 (4): 452–460.

Peatling, S. (2008) 'Centrelink smothered by "infractions"', *The Sydney Morning Herald*, January 15—http://www.smh.com.au/news/national/centrelink-smothered-by-infrac...

Pech, J. (1997) 'Voice, Choice and Contract: Customer Focus in Programs for Unemployed People', *Department of Social Security Policy Discussion Paper No. 9*, Australian Government Printing Service.

Penglase, J. (2005) *Orphans of the Living: Growing up in 'care' in twentieth-century Australia*, Fremantle: Curtin University Books with Fremantle Arts Centre Press.

Perrow, C. (1986) 'Economic Theories of Organization', *Theory and Society*, 15, 11–45.

Pettit, P. (1997) *Republicanism: a Theory of Freedom and Government*, Oxford: Oxford University Press.

Pettit, P. (2002) 'Keeping Republican Freedom Simple: on a difference with Quentin Skinner', *Political Theory*, 30: 3, 339–357.

Pilgrim, D. and L. Waldron (1998) 'User involvement in mental health service development: How far can it go?', *Journal of Mental Health*, 7 (1), 95–104.

Pilgrim, D. and A. Rogers (1999) 'Mental Health Policy and the Politics of Mental Health: a three tier analytical framework', *Policy and Politics*, 27 (1), 13–25.

Race, K., E. Wakeford and D. McInnes (1999) '"Taking medicine" and the clinical encounter', Paper presented at the 10th Conference on Social Aspects of AIDS, South Bank University, London, June.

Race, K. and E. Wakeford (2000) 'Dosing on time: developing adherent practice with highly active anti-retroviral therapy', *Culture, Health & Sexuality*, 2 (2), 213–228.

Race, K., D. McInnes, E. Wakeford, V. Kleinert, M. McMurchie and M. Kidd (2001) *Adherence and Communication: Reports from a study of HIV general practice*, University of New South Wales: National Centre in HIV Social Research, Monograph 8.

Raphael, B. (2005) 'Grief, Trauma and Who We Are', *Dialogue*, Academy of the Social Sciences of Australia, 24 (3), 31–46.

Riessman, F. (1984) 'The New Consumer Revolution: From Protection to Empowerment', *Social Policy*, Summer, 2–3.

Rodman, F. (2003) *Winnicott: Life and Work*, Cambridge, MA: Perseus Books.

Ronalds, C. (1989) *I'm Still an Individual'. A Blueprint for the Rights of Residents in Nursing Homes and Hostels,* Issues Paper, Department of Community Services and Health, Canberra.

Rose, N. (1999) 'Freedom', in *Powers of Freedom: Reframing political thought*, Cambridge: Cambridge University Press, 61–98.

Rosengarten, M., K. Race and S. Kippax (2000) *'Touch wood, everything will be ok': gay men's understandings of clinical markers in sexual practice*, Monograph 7, University of New South Wales: National Centre in HIV Social Research.

Ross, S. (2003) 'Customer Experience Management: Serving the Citizen Better in Centrelink', *Canberra Bulletin of Public Administration*, 106, 21–4.

Rothfield, P. (1997) Menopausal Embodiment, in P. Komesaroff, P. Rothfield and J. Daly (eds) *Reinterpreting Menopause: Cultural and Philosophical Issues.* New York and London: Routledge.

Rowe, M. and G. Dowsett (2008) 'Sex, love, friendship, belonging and place: is there a role for "gay community" in HIV prevention today?', *Culture, Health and Sexuality*, 11, 329–344.

Rowlands, D. (1999) 'Purchaser-provider in Social Policy Delivery: Prolegomena to an Evaluation of the Centrelink Arrangements', in S. Shaver and P. Saunders (eds) *Social Policy for the 21st Century: Justice and Responsibility, Proceedings of the National Social Policy Conference, Volume 2*, Sydney 21–23 July, University of New South Wales: Social Policy Research Centre, 221–241.

Roy, A. (2001) 'Contracts in Close Personal Relationships', Prepared for the Law Commission of Canada, Montreal, June 25.

Saunders, P. (2005) 'Disability, Poverty and Living Standards: Reviewing Australian Evidence and Policies', SPRC Discussion Paper No. 145, December, University of New South Wales: The Social Policy Research Centre.

Sax, S. (1985) *A Strife of Interests. Politics and Policies in Australian Health Services*, Sydney, George Allen and Unwin.

Sayce, L. (2003) 'Beyond Good Intentions: Making Anti-discrimination Strategies Work', *Disability & Society*, 18: 5, 625–642.

Scharf, T. and C.G. Wenger (eds) (1995) *International Perspectives on Community Care of Older People*, Aldershot: Avebury.

Scourfield, P. (2005) 'Implementing the Community Care (Direct Payments) Act: Will the Supply of Personal Assistants meet the Demand and at what Price?', *Journal of Social Policy*, 34 (3), 469–488.

Scourfield, P. (2006) "What matters is what works"? How discourses of modernization have both silenced and limited debate on domiciliary care for older people, *Critical Social Policy* 26 (1), 5–30.

Scourfield, P. (2007) 'Social Care and the Modern Citizen: Client, Consumer, Service User, Manager and Entrepreneur', *British Journal of Social Work*, 37, 107–122.

Seabury, B. (1976) 'The Contract: Use, Abuses, and Limitations', *Social Work*, 2 (1), 16–24.

Shaddock, A. and P. Bramston (1991) 'Individual Service Plans: The Policy-Practice Gap', *Australian and New Zealand of Developmental Disabilities*, 17 (1), 73–81.

Shaddock, A., S. Guggenheimer, M. Rawlings and E. Bugel (1993) 'Having Your Say: Perceptions of Self-Advocates on the Involvement of People with an Intellectual Disability on Decisions About their Lives', *Australian Disability Review*, 2 (93): 45–54.

Sheets-Johnstone, M. (1999) *The Primacy of Movement*, Amsterdam/Philadelphia: John Benjamins Publishing Company.

Shuda, S. and Just Anna (2007) 'Finding a way towards being', in C. Flaskas, I. McCarthy and J. Sheehan (eds) *Hope and Despair in Narrative and Family Therapy*, London and New York: Routledge, 87–100.

Siegel, D. (1999) *The Developing Mind: How Relationships and the Brain Interact to Shape Who We Are*, New York and London: The Guildford Press.

Siegel, D. (2007) *The Mindful Brain: Reflection and Attunement in the Cultivation of Well-being*, New York and London: W.W. Norton.

Sinason, V. (1992) *Mental Handicap and the Human Condition: New Approaches from the Tavistock*, London: Free Association Books.

Skinner, Q. (1998) *Liberty Before Liberalism*, Cambridge: Cambridge University Press.

South Australian Department for Correctional Services (1994) *Annual Report 1993–1994*, Adelaide: Government of South Australia.

South Australian Department for Correctional Services (1995) *Annual Report 1994–1995*, Adelaide: Adelaide: Government of South Australia.

South Australian Department for Correctional Services (1996) *Annual Report 1995–1996*, Adelaide: Adelaide: Government of South Australia.

South Australian Department for Correctional Services (1998) *Annual Report 1997–1998*, Adelaide: Adelaide: Government of South Australia.

South Australian Department for Correctional Services (1999) *Annual Report 1998–1999*, Adelaide: Adelaide: Government of South Australia.

Stanley, N. (1999) 'User-Practitioner Transactions in the New Culture of Community Care', *British Journal of Social Work*, 29, 417–435.

Steyaert, J. (1997) 'Peeling the client information systems onion', in N. Gould and K. Moultrie (eds) *Effective policy, planning and implementation: information management in social services*, Aldershot: Avebury; 27–47.

Stojkovic, S. and M. Farkas (2003) *Correctional Leadership: A Cultural Perspective*, Melbourne, Australia: Thomson Wadsworth.

SWAG (1982) *Abuse of the Elderly. A report on the results of a phone-in study of elder abuse,* Social Welfare Action Group, C/- Department of Social Work, University of Sydney, Sydney.

The LAC Project Australia (2004) *Newsletter*, March.

The LAC Project Australia (2004) *Newsletter*, August.

Tregeagle, S. and L. Treleaven (2006) 'Key questions in considering guided practice for vulnerable Australian children', *Australian Journal of Social Issues*, 41 (3), 359–369.

Tully, J. (1980) *A Discourse on Property: John Locke and his Adversaries*, Cambridge: Cambridge University Press.

Tully, J. (1993) *An Approach to Political Philosophy: Locke in Contexts*, Cambridge: Cambridge University Press.

Ungerson, C. (1997) 'Give Them the Money: Is Cash a Route to Empowerment?', *Social Policy & Administration*, 31 (1), 45–53.

Vardon, S. (1997) 'Are Prisoners Clients?', *Australian Journal of Public Administration*, 56 (1), 127–141.

Vardon, S. (1999a) 'Meeting the challenge: promoting inclusion, redressing exclusion in service delivery', Presentation to the 26th Annual Conference, The Australian Association of Social Workers, Brisbane, Queensland, 28th September.

Vardon, S. (1999b) 'Creating a Customer Service Culture for a national government', Address given at the International Summit on Public Service Reform, Winnipeg, Manitoba, 10 June.

Vardon, S. (2000) 'One-to-One: The Art of Personalised Service', Presentation to the 3rd Annual Conference, The Case Management Society of Australia, University of Melbourne, 11 February.

Vardon, S. (2003) 'Moving Service Delivery Forward: The Practical and the Tactical—The Centrelink Experience Australia', PowerPoint slides, presented in Canada (provided to author by Sue Vardon).

Varela, F., E. Thompson and E. Rosch (1993) *The Embodied Mind: Cognitive Science and Human Experience*, Cambridge, Mass. and London, England: MIT Press.

Ward, H. (1998) 'Using a child development model to assess the outcomes of social work interventions with families', *Children & Society*, 12 (3), 202–211.

Ward, T. and C. Stewart (2003) 'Criminogenic Needs and Human Needs: a Theoretical Model', *Psychology, Crime & Law*, 9 (2), 125–143.

Ward, T. and A. Birgden (2007) Human Rights and Correctional Clinical Practice, *Aggression and Violent Behavior*, doi:10.1016/j.avb2007.05.001. [online] Available at: www.sciencedirect.com

Ward, T. and B. Marshall (2007) Narrative Identity and Offender Rehabilitation, *International Journal of Offender Therapy and Comparative Criminology*, 51 (3), 279–297.

Warnes, A., L. Warren and M. Nolan (2000) 'Health, Welfare and Old Age: Transformations and Critiques', in A. Warnes, L. Warren and M. Nolan (eds) *Care Services for Later Life: Transformations and Critiques*, London and Philadelphia: Jessica Kingsley Publishers.

Welch, M. (1996) *Corrections: A Critical Approach*, New York: USA, McGraw-Hill Companies.

Weller, P. (1997) 'Are Prisoners Clients?', *Australian Journal of Public Administration*, 56: 1, 125–127.

Westacott, R. (n.d.) 'HIV-positive community: a thing of the past?', Australian Federation of AIDS Organisations (AFAO)—www.afao.org.au/view_articles.asp

Whitehead, P., T. Ward and R. Collie (2007) 'Time for a Change: Applying the Good Lives Model of Rehabilitation to a High-Risk Violent Offender', *International Journal of Offender Therapy and Comparative Criminology*, 1–21.

Wightman, J. (2000) 'Intimate Relationships, Relational Contract Theory and the Reach of Contract', *Feminist Legal Studies*, 8: 93–131.

Wilenski, P. (1986) *Public Power & Public Administration*, Sydney: Hale & Iremonger.

Williams, F. (1999) 'Good Enough Principles for Welfare', *Journal of Social Policy*, 28: 4, 667–687.

Williams, F. (2000) 'Travels with Nanny, Destination Good Enough. A Personal/Intellectual Journey through the Welfare State', Inaugural Lecture 11 May 2000, University of Leeds—[online] Available at: http://www.leeds.ac.uk/sociology/inaugural/

Winnicott, C. (1989) 'D.W.W.: A Reflection', in D. Winnicott *Psychoanalytic Explorations*, C. Winnicott, R. Shepherd and M. Davis (eds), London: Karnac, 1–21.

Winnicott, D. (1986) 'Some thoughts on the meaning of the word "Democracy"', in *Home Is Where We Start From*, Penguin Books, 239–260.
Winnicott, D. (1989a) *Psychoanalytic Explorations*, C. Winnicott, R. Shepherd, and M. Davis (eds), London: Karnac.
Winnicott, D. (1989b) *Playing & Reality*, London and New York: Routledge.
Winnicott, D. (1990) 'The Theory of the Parent-Infant Relationship', in *The Maturational Processes and the Facilitating Environment*, London: Karnac, 37–56.
Winnicott, D. (1991a) 'Hate in the Counter-Transference', in *Through Paediatrics to Psychoanalysis: Collected Papers*, London: Karnac, 194–204.
Winnicott, D. (1991b) 'Mind and its Relation to the Psyche-Soma' in *Through Paediatrics to Psychoanalysis: Collected Papers*, London: Karnac, 243–255.
Wirth, W. (1991) 'Responding to Citizens Needs: From Bureaucratic Accountability to Individual Coproduction in the Public Sector', in F.-X. Kaufman (ed.) *The Public Sector: Challenge for Coordination and Learning*, Berlin and New York: De Gruyter.
Wise, S. (2003) 'An Evaluation of a Trial of Looking After Children in the State of Victoria, Australia', *Children & Society*, 17, 3–17.
Wolfensberger, W. (1972) *Normalization. The principle of normalization in human services*, Toronto, National Institute on Mental Retardation.
Woodroofe, K. (1962) *From Charity to Social Work In England and the United States*, London: Routledge & Kegan Paul.
Yeatman, A. (1989) *Review of Domiciliary Care Services in South Australia: Final Report*, South Australia: State Print.
Yeatman, A. (1990) *Bureaucrats, Technocrats, Femocrats: Essays on the Contemporary Australian State*, Sydney, Wellington, London and Boston: Allen & Unwin.
Yeatman, A. (1998a) 'Activism and the Policy Process', in A. Yeatman (ed.) *Activism and the Policy Process*, St Leonards NSW: Allen & Unwin, 16–36.
Yeatman, A. (1998b) 'Interpreting Contemporary Contractualism', in M. Dean and B. Hindess (eds) *Governing Australia: Studies in Contemporary Rationalities of Government*, Cambridge: Cambridge University Press, 227–242.
Yeatman, A. (2000) 'Mutual Obligation: what kind of contract is this?', in P. Saunders (ed.) *Reforming the Australian Welfare State, Melbourne: Australian Institute of Family Studies*, Commonwealth of Australia, 156–177.
Yeatman, A. (2001) 'Who is the subject of human rights?', in D. Meredyth and J. Minson (eds) *Citizenship and Cultural Policy*, London, Thousand Oaks and New Delhi: Sage, 104–120.
Yeatman, A. (2004) 'Social Policy, Freedom and Individuality', *Australian Journal of Public Administration* 63: 4, 80–90.
Yeatman, A. (2007a) 'Varieties of Individualism', in C. Howard (ed.) *Contested Individualization: Debates about Contemporary Personhood*, New York and Basingstoke: Palgrave Macmillan, 45–61.
Yeatman, A. (2007b) 'The Subject of Citizenship', *Citizenship Studies* 11: 1, 105–116.
Yeatman, A. (2007c) 'Freedom and the Feldenkrais Method', *IFF Academy Feldenkrais Research Journal* 2006/2007 Vol. 3 (online edition).
Yeatman, A. (2009) 'Self-preservation and the Idea of the State', in A. Yeatman, K. Stullerova and M. Zolkos (eds) *State, Security and Subject Formation*, New York: Continuum.
Yeatman, A. and J. Penglase (2004) 'Looking After Children: a case of individualized service delivery', *Australian Journal of Social Issues* 39 (3), 233–248.

Young, D. and R. Quibell (2000) 'Why Rights are Never Enough: rights, intellectual disability and understanding', *Disability & Society*, 15 (5), 747–764.

Young, I. (1997) 'Asymmetrical Reciprocity: on moral respect, wonder and enlarged thought', in *Intersecting Voices: Dilemmas of gender, Political Philosophy, and Policy*, Princeton: Princeton University Press, 38–60.

Young, I. (2000) 'Inclusive Political Communication', in *Inclusion and Democracy*, Oxford: Oxford University Press.

Zanetti, C. (1998) 'Managing Change: Focus on Improving Service Quality and Information Management', *Australian Journal of Public Administration*, 57 (4), 3–13.

Index

abuse, 37, 38–9, 58
  child, 38, 143–4, *see also* Looking
    After Children (LAC) Initiative
  child sexual, 21–2, 37
  sexual, 22
  'systems abuse', 27, 142, 144
    (Table 9.1), 144–5, 245
activism, gay community, 188–90,
    191, 193, 195, 207–8, n. 209,
    see also HIV-AIDS
aged care, *see* care, community aged
Aged Care Act (1997), 172
Aged Care Reform Strategy, 168–9
agency theory, 139
Ainsworth, Frank, 143–4, 146
Alvarez, Anne, 17, 43–4, 65–6
'Anna', *see* 'Just Anna'
Arendt, Hannah, 70–1, 77
Aristotle, 5, 84
Australasian Society for HIV Medicine
    (ASHM), 193, 194, 196–7, 208
Australian Federation of AIDS
    Organisations, 189

Barnardos Australia, 142, 145–7, 148,
    150–5, 156, 163, n. 164, *see also*
    Looking After Children (LAC)
    Initiative
Beck, Allen, 239
Benevolent Society, 166, 176–7, n. 185,
    see also care, community aged *and*
    Help at Home service
Benjamin, Jessica, 89, 98, 99–103
Beresford, Peter, 78
Berg, Insoo Kim, 105–7
Bick, Esther, 32
Bigby, Christine, n. 87
Bion, Wilfred, 32, 65, 70
Blackstone, Sir William, 13
Bollas, Christopher, 49, 58, 64–7, 71,
    n. 72, 91
Bowlby, John, 32, 36–7
Braithwaite, John, 61

Bramston, Paul, 231
breastfeeding, 59–60
British Poor Law (1834), 15, 34, 35–6
British Report on the Working Party
    of Social Workers in the Local
    Authority Health and Welfare
    Services (1959), n. 40
Brown, David, 240
bureaucracy, public, 119–40
  ethos of, 125–8
  see also individualization *and* welfare
    services, consumer model of

care
  community, 74–6, n. 88, 169,
    175–6, 183
  community aged, 165–85
  home-based, 168–9, 172, 174, 177–84
  individualized, 170–4
  institutional, 74–5, 167–9, 176–7
  out-of-home, 141–64, 245
  palliative, 39, 92–3
  person-centred, 90–4
  personal, 17–18, 211–12
  see also Help at Home service *and*
    hostels *and* institutionalization
    and welfare services, consumer
    model of
Carlson, Peter, 239
Carnaby, Steven, 231
case management, *see* correctional
    services, case management
Cashmore, Judy, 143–4, 146
Centrelink, 119–40, 242, 245
  creation of, 119–25
  customer service and, 128–31
  ethos of, 120–8, 135–8
  internal organization of, 135–8
  personalized service and, 134–5
  service delivery, 132–4
  see also policy, social *and* Vardon,
    Sue *and* welfare services,
    consumer model of

self, 25–40, 49–50, 90–4
  independence of, 64, 67–9
  integrity of, 64–7
  as subject of welfare, 7–12, 17–19,
    22–3, 25, 42–9, 63–71
self-awareness, 29–30, 33, 38, 64,
    69–71
self-government, 5, 14
self-image, 29
self-preservation, 6–7, 10, 12–14, 22,
    n. 23, 25, 34, 40, 51–2, 79, 93
sexual abuse, *see* abuse, sexual
Shaddock, Ann, 231
shell-shock, 35–6
Shuda, Suzanne, 95–8, 105
Sinason, Valerie, 39, 53–5, 68
Singh, Gurnam, 78–9
Skinner, Quentin, 51
slavery, 52, 54, 55, 96
social security, 34, *compare* welfare
    and welfare services
social policy, *see* policy, social
Socrates, 70–1
space
  jurisdictional, 56
  relational, 56–61
state, the 19–23, 34, 42, 55, 58–61,
    128
  and the law, 60–1
  as public authority, 56, 128
  public life and, 47–8, 55
  see also welfare state
status, 3, 38, 52, 60–1, 64, 92
  citizenship and, 33
  individualization and, 3
subject
  as embodied self, 28–33, 34, 39
  of freedom, 4–5
  of right, 3, 6, 7–8, 13, 34, 35, 40,
    42–56, 64, 94
  as self, 7, 9–12, 14–15, 16, 17–19,
    22–3, 25, 42–4, 56–7, 63–71
  of will, 4–5, 7–8, 14–15, 16, 19, 26,
    42–4, 56–7, 81–3
subjectivity, 18, 25, 32–3, 35, 37,
    38–9, 42–56, 64–6, 83, 86, 90–1
  inter-subjectivity, 46–8, 89, 97–101,
    102, 107, 112
subjective right, *see* right, subjective

Tavistock Institute, 30, *see also*
    psychoanalysis
trauma, 35–6, 37, 45, 48, 54–5
Tustin, Frances, 32

unemployment, 48

Vardon, Sue, 104–5, 120, 121–6,
    129–31, 132–40, 235–6, 237,
    241–51

Wallbridge, 59, n. 61, n. 62
Ward, Tony, 237
Weber, Max, 127–8
Welch, Michael, 239
welfare
  advocacy of, 25–7, 98–9, 143–5,
    n. 185
  contestation of, 12–19, 35
  debate, 5, 15, 22–3, 26
  the deliverer, and; *see* welfare
    professionals
  ethos of, 34–5, 109, 119–25,
    151–3
  government and, 18–23, 25, 74–5,
    81, 110–16, 119–25, 175–6,
    221, 232–3
  reform, 15–16, 143–5, 241–57:
    Australian, *see* correctional
    services, reform of, South
    Australia (1993–1997); U.S.
    (1990s), 15–16
  resources and, 22, 79–80
  self-preservation and, 6, 47–8
  self as subject of, 22–3, 26, 63–71,
    89, 92–4
  will as subject of, 22–3, 39–40, 43,
    73–87
  see also bureaucracy, public *and*
    Centrelink *and* welfare
    services
welfare professional, 8, 17–19, 20, 21,
    26–7, 38–9, 43–6, 52–5, 59, 75,
    78–9, 93, 97–104, 112–15, 151–3,
    174, 179–84, 210–13, 217–18,
    221–31, 247–9, 255–7
  ethics of, 26–7
  sense of self and, 19, 89, 90, 108–9
  as will, 81